FROM
KNOW-HOW
TO
NOWHERE

FROM
KNOW-HOW
TO
NOWHERE

The Development
of American Technology

ELTING E. MORISON

Basic Books, Inc., Publishers

NEW YORK

T
21
M7
1975

Library of Congress Cataloging in Publication Data

Morison, Elting Elmore.
From know-how to nowhere.

Bibliography: p.
1. Technology—History—United States. I. Title.
T21.M7   609'.73   74-79279
ISBN 0-465-02580-3

Copyright © 1974 by Basic Books, Inc.
Library of Congress Catalog Card Number: 74-79279
ISBN: 0-465-02580-3
Printed in the United States of America
DESIGNED BY VINCENT TORRE
74 75 76 77   10 9 8 7 6 5 4 3 2 1

TO E.F.M. AND S.S.C.

"Works themselves are of greater value as pledges of truth than as contributing to the comforts of life."

—Francis Bacon

"They acquire the habit of always considering themselves as standing alone and they are apt to imagine that their whole destiny is in their own hands."

—Alexis de Tocqueville

"The business of the future is dangerous."

—A. N. Whitehead

PREFACE

A FRIEND of mine, a man of science, finds my idea that the narrative can be a form of thought hilarious. I do not propose to argue the point here; it is mentioned only because it explains something about the structure of this book. My interest in what might be done with the future comes out of a much longer engagement with the past. Hence there is, in these pages, a good deal of history and therefore of narration.

The history deals with how we have built or made certain kinds of things and how we have decided what to build or make. There is, in a way, not much that is new in these historical accounts. Most of the material is easily available. But since it deals with matters—canals, locomotives, steel ingots, electric light bulbs—which until very recently were not believed to be a necessary part of our learning, indeed were often assumed to be culturally inappropriate, not many people have paid much attention to it. In that sense I hope it will be new to many of those who may read these pages. Also I

hope that the information has been put in the service of a line
of thought that may give it novel force.

At the end of this line of thought is a suggested way to
give the future a shape consonant with our needs and best intentions. I am told that it is a modest proposal. That may be
because, in searching for means to deal with current difficulties, it starts somewhere near the bottom rather than somewhere near the top—or more accurately, it begins with
small pieces rather than the big picture. What may happen when the sights are set on the big picture was nicely
revealed in the deliberations of a conference I recently attended on what to do about what was then the most obvious
dysfunction in our system—the energy crisis. The engineers
said it was a matter for improved technology, the economists said it was a matter of pricing, the officials of government said it was a matter of increasing and centralizing authority, perhaps a Czar or at least a Cabinet member, those
in industry said it was, on the whole, a matter of capital and
tax structures. At the tail end there was a session given over
to "life styles"—which is a term designed, one assumes, to so
denature the topic of values that one can bear to discuss it at
all. At this time a paper was read that advocated the development of a society that would be based on growing things.

The mix of members in that conference reflected a current
truth. In any society based on technology every important
situation contains almost everything from the second law of
thermodynamics to the way, depending on conditions of
labor, transport, and communication, of a wight with a
maid. Start from the siting of a power plant, the internal
combustion engine, or the double helix, and one comes in
time upon the interrelated ordinances of nature, man, and
God. Within the systems of technology we have devised to
take the place of the natural world everything connects—or
should be made to do so.

But the results of the discussions of the various members of the conference as they talked past each other were not reassuring. Those with 20/20 visual acuity in their own fields, on being presented with a whole elephant, seemed to do no better with their tunneled vision than had the blind men before them.

The modest proposal offered in these pages suggests a means for bringing together all interested parties—including those who don't know much but have a stake in the game because whatever happens happens to them—at the point of actual decision in particular cases that represent the general workings of the systems of technology. It suggests a way that all the requisite information—technical, economic, political, social, aesthetic—can be collected, organized, and put to the interested parties for their collective analysis, interpretation, and ultimate choice. It suggests a method for negotiating, from evidence held in common, understandings that will give accommodation, in due proportion, to all the conflicting interests in a situation. The hope is that it also suggests how those values which are expressions of our best intentions toward each other (as opposed to what is merely personally comforting—as in a life style) may be recognized and put to work in the design and regulation of the mechanical operations that are supposed to increase our comfort.

As already stated, each situation—power plant, engine, double helix—seems, if diligently investigated, to contain all the essential ingredients of the time. And if such investigations are pursued to the end one comes always upon the same question. Whether the situations develop from the derangement of the atmosphere, the sense that natural resources have finite limits, the exponential increase in the rate of change in mechanical systems, the anticipated power of computers to overorganize things, or the foreboded power of medicine to control the organization of our personalities—they all come down to the question of whether men can handle the knowledge they have acquired and the machines they have built.

The tendency, in the search for proper handling, is to increase and concentrate power and to sharpen further the wits of the expert. All history suggests that neither authority nor the mind is sufficient if it works outside a restraining context of general purpose. Recent history suggests that a context built only upon considerations of efficiency within the technical systems that enclose us is also insufficient. It is the hope that from the recurring exercises in particular cases as here proposed men may learn enough about their machinery and themselves to invent in time a context—a general purpose—that will take into account what both machines and men need to keep running in good order.

I am in the debt of several institutions and many men and women for aid and comfort in the writing of this book. Some years ago I went to one of the service academies to give a talk. On arrival I was told that the first, great, and indeed only commandment was to keep the cadets awake. They called the magnificent hall to which they went to receive instruction from those in the outside world the Master Bedroom. So I threw away a prepared text and took them on with the forces of anecdote recollected in some trepidation. Most of the stories were taken from the history of the United States Navy in the years from 1865 to 1890. That was a strange time. There was, for instance, a secretary of the navy who was astounded to discover that ships were hollow and men-of-war often took target practice by firing away at targets that were not there. So I had not much trouble finding funny things that had happened on the way to Manila Bay. Working along through these engaging anecdotes, I came upon the idea that supplies the substance of Chapter Eight and served both as a point of departure and an organizing principle for the development of this book.

Last year I was invited to give the Messenger Lectures at Cornell University. In preparation for this appearance I did most of the investigation on which my description of early American engineering projects depends. From my discussions with my hosts in Ithaca, members of the Program on Science, Technology, and Society, I learned much that increased my understanding of the study I was engaged in.

The generous terms of my appointment at the Massachusetts Institute of Technology greatly facilitated both the research and the writing. From my long association with members of the faculty of this exciting institution I have derived whatever understanding of the intellectual processes of science and engineering may be discerned in this book.

I am also deeply in the debt of Perri Beth Irvings, who for one year bore a major share in the task of historical research. My colleagues D. Quinn Mills and Sir William Hawthorne read the manuscript, as did my brothers, Dr. Robert S. Morison and John H. Morison. Each offered correction and stimulating comment from which these pages greatly profit. By now all those things, ancillary and fundamental, that wives can do to help their husbands write a book have been fully described in prefaces like this. Elizabeth Forbes Morison did them all in a way that made me feel she really wanted to.

Peterborough,   ELTING E. MORISON
New Hampshire

CONTENTS

PART I

The Rule of Thumb

PART II

Ideas Come to Power

PART

I

The Rule of Thumb

CHAPTER 1

Some Introductory Remarks

THE LINE of argument in this book goes like this: We can now build machines that will do almost everything for us from cooling a room in the heat of summer to blowing up the world. We can arrange these devices in technical systems that in their operation profoundly modify and sometimes take the place of our natural environment. The workings of these systems, if insufficiently controlled, certainly contaminate and may in time exhaust significant resources of nature. They may well, also, create conditions that human beings, with all their powers of adaptation, cannot tolerate—at least cannot tolerate without the loss of qualities and authorities that have been assumed to be essential characteristics of human being.

The task at hand is to design the pieces of machinery and the structure of the enclosing systems to prevent such things from happening. Put more positively, it is to design and control things so that the artificial surrounding we create for ourselves will serve our interests better than the supplanted natural environment did.

This, in a way, is what Antiphon had in mind when he said two thousand years ago, "Mastered by Nature, we o'ercome by Art." But he did not foresee the day when the power in the machinery and the inertia in the systems would be so great that we might be mastered by the products of that Art; hoisted, as it were, by our own ingenious petards. How to give these products an appropriate order—that is, how to organize a technological world we can live in—is now the great question.

The criteria for such design and control cannot be established by a search for the maximum potential in each particular machine or system—how better to cool a room; how more easily to blow up some part of the world we do not, at the moment, want. The criteria must derive from some general scheme that all the parts and pieces can fit into and serve. Such a scheme cannot be based only on our knowledge of what machines can be built to do, which is almost anything. It has to be grounded in the sense of ourselves as the governing reference point. The controlling factor in the design problem is what we take the human condition to be.

Nature, to be commanded, must be obeyed. That great imperative has guided the investigation of the external world for almost four hundred years. It must now be applied to the investigations of our own nature. For if we are to control the technological world we are building, we must first command ourselves, and that command rests upon our understanding of, and respect for, the fundamental organization of our being.

In the building of any new world, it is probably simpler, as in the first creation, to start out when things are without form, and void. Then the dry land and the two great lights and the herb-yielding seed and the creeping things can be put in when and where the spirit moves. And it would certainly be easier for us if, as on the first occasion, we could come in to take our place among the given conditions as a sort of divine afterthought. But we are already here as a first cause and prime mover. And, to repeat, if we are to build a new firmament fit for us to live in out of the materials and forces now available, our first order of business is to develop a knowledge of ourselves, and a respect for ourselves, certain enough to enable us to build a technological firmament that will really fit us.

That, together with some supplementary suggestions and proposals, is the main line of argument in this book. It is put forward here at the outset because it may take some time to get to it. Much that follows is simply history, and history with its extending linear progression is not the most economical way to get at a subject. But how we got to where we are is, in its way, as interesting as what we might do now that we are here. And some feeling for what was done before may help in deciding what to do next.

Since men have been making things for a long time, one could start way back—at least as far back as the waterworks in Mesopotamia in the time of Tiglath Pileser I. In these pages, the narrative is severely foreshortened. The evidence of history will be presented through the description of the work of a handful of men who, at different times, built and made things in this country. Taken all together, their lives and labors span the years from 1800 to the present. The narrative starts at a point where men found they did not know how to construct a small lock in a short canal designed to join Wood Creek with the Mohawk River in upstate New York. It ends in the present, when we have, among other things, put men on the moon.

There is obviously a considerable advance in competence here. As a developing process, this impressive change can stand almost self-contained within the longer reaches of the history of technology. The 175 years can be taken in fact as a microcosm, a small fraction that contains, not the detailed record, but in its condensed form, the essential meaning of the whole history. Anyone who understands what happened in this country after 1800 understands sufficiently the dynamics of engineering development through the ages. Before getting to a closer examination of this period, it may be useful to yield momentarily to the historian's temptation to put the matter in a little larger perspective.

At the center of all engineering lies the problem of converting knowledge into practice. It is a very complicated process. Part of that problem is simply the timeless difficulty of translating the abstract into the real and the general into a particular that really works. And part of it, equally timeless, is the clouded connection between knowing and doing. Each feeds off the other with varying appetite. For instance, what is called the state of the art is taken to reflect what one can do at any given moment, but it is also a decisive expression of what is known and not known at the time. Furthermore, refinements of technique—of ways of doing things—may appear to be, and sometimes are, dramatic improvements in the state of the art, but fundamental advances derive only from increases in the amount of information available. Sometimes these increases are produced by the searches of those who simply want to know more; sometimes by those who force the search because they want to do something better—or different. In any case, the long-run result is always the same. While men, as W. G. Sumner said, begin with acts not ideas, the spring behind enlarging action is, in the end, further knowledge and thought. That, in a way, is what the history of engineering is all about.

The Romans, both in what they did and did not do, nicely demonstrate these points. They built, as everyone knows, a remarkable set of structures: roads, aqueducts, temples, arenas, mine shafts, sewage disposals, bridges, municipal waterworks. In the course of this construction, they learned to make and use a varied set of instruments: pulleys, pumps, hoists, levels, cranes, hydraulic cement, metal trusses, and even rivets. In their greatest period, one hundred years either side of the Crucifixion, they built great structures from Asia Minor to the British Isles. Some of these still stand in distinctive grandeur as monuments to the genius of their creators.

It is a sobering thought that the Coliseum, built to fill the same need as Shea Stadium or the Astrodome, has lasted two thousand years. It is far more remarkable, however, that the methods used by the Romans in their building endured for almost as long. For this, a man named Marcus Vetruvius Pollio is at least in part responsible. He lived in the time of Caesar Augustus and was a superintendent of *ballistae* (machines for hurling heavy weights) and other military engines. He was also an architect, and like most architects in those days, he put his hand to building anything that could be made of brick and stone.

Somewhere around 20 B.C., he published a book called *De architectura libra decem*. This work contains some not very interesting summaries of Greek descriptions of how the Greeks had built things. What was more interesting and much more useful was the author's explanations of what he had learned on the job. The volume became a textbook on Roman engineering.

Fifteen hundred years later, Bramante, Michelangelo, Palladio, and the other great builders of the Renaissance took Vetruvius as their chief authority. "In every point," it has been said, "his precepts were accepted as final." It was quite a run for an unrevised textbook. And what the men of the Renaissance learned from *De architectura*, they passed on to those who came after them. So what the Romans knew about foundations, concrete, timber piling, hoists, pile drivers, and bearing arches was passed on down through the ages. To the time of the first steam engine, what the Romans had done was, in many areas of engineering, a standard to repair to.

This extraordinary state of affairs is not to be attributed, of course, to the irresistible authority of Vetruvius. The important cause was that for eighteen centuries the materials and forces men worked with remained fairly fixed—timber, stone, wind, falling water, animal energy. The Romans, within this continuing context, become especially interesting for two reasons. First, it seems on the whole true that in brick and stone none who followed them during eighteen hundred years did better work. Early on, they had pushed the state of the art, within the given conditions, almost to its farthest limits. Even in design. Here they moved steadily, as James Finch points out, toward the organization of their materials and forces with maximum economy and grace.

As evidence of this progress, he cites the difference between the Pont du Gard built in southern France in the first years of the Christian era, and the aqueduct in Segovia, Spain, constructed a century later. Both still stand. In the massive loom of the former, there is a sense of "over design." In the airy lines of the latter, there is "a daring elegance," which is, it might be said, the ultimate morality of the engineer—if it works.

The Roman record demonstrates how much can be learned from experience—doing work. It also suggests the limits imposed on the understanding if one learns primarily by doing. Practice, supported only by the knowledge obtained from practice, tends to stay in the same place. The Romans cared little, in fact, for the general implications of their work; they rarely sought the reasons for things or tried to build a sustaining structure of theory around what they were doing.

The same was true of those who followed them for a great many years. So with a fixed set of resources and a stable body of procedures, the art remained, for a long time, in a fairly steady state. It was only in the early seventeenth century that men working with these same materials and forces began in a general way to feel the need to extend what Francis Bacon called "useful knowledge" about the natural world. Then things began to happen.

The connections between doing and knowing and understanding and thinking vary with the occasion and are, as already suggested, at all times complicated. Since these varying connections supply much of the structure for the narrative which follows, a little more may be said about them by way of introduction here.

If it is true that men begin with acts, it is also true that they start looking for knowledge almost immediately. Indeed, the history of Western culture—or a great part of it—can be written from the very beginning simply as a search for further information. In the first chapters of Genesis, the first thing the first human beings did was to try to find out more than they, at their creation, knew. If the Bible is one of the keys to the way we look at life, the Greek spirit is the other. And the Greeks set knowing above all things. As John H. Randall said, "They could be moved strongly by nothing they did not understand—[and they] searched heaven and earth for the reasons for things."

Why are men inquiring creatures? What lies at the bottom of the zeal to learn? For such questions, there may be only dusty answers. It is said in Genesis that the Lord God was put out by the eating of the fruit because, in so doing, "the man is become as one of us." Somewhat later, Socrates took the position that learning was the end of life because "no one is allowed to enter the company of the gods but the lovers of knowledge only."

In both cases, the point seems to have been that by learning men could associate with those who were in authority because they knew everything. In any event, the belief seems established at the very beginning that what made men different from, indeed superior to, all other living things was the ability to acquire and process information. And, from the beginning, that ability was used in efforts to make men, the universe, and the place of men in that vast universe more intelligible.

Sometimes, as in the Bible, these efforts at increased intelligibility were worked out in precise and concrete detail and in the narrative form. Later, beginning especially with the Greeks, they were cast in the abstract, often in mathematics, and in the shape of rather grand concepts. Because at the start, and for a good many succeeding centuries, not much of all there was to know was in fact known, it was necessary in the interest of comprehensiveness to fill in the vacancies in the narrative with fictions or mystical perceptions and to support thin parts in the concepts with myths or metaphysics.

The knowledge thus acquired and organized served some very useful purposes. That which had to do with man supplied the underpinning for certain regulatory schemes in the ordering of human affairs—conventions, customs, laws, codes of the moral, ethical, and chivalric. That which had to do with the universe enabled men to give increasingly clear, if often mistaken, descriptions of the nature of their physical surroundings. Thus, moving slowly out of mystery into defined conditions, they could proceed with growing confidence to and fro in their world.

For a long time, this restless search for further information rested primarily on speculation and had to do principally with the largest questions of life—the nature of reality, the meaning of existence, and what to do to be saved, if not in this world at least in the next. It had very little to do with simplifying the day's work. For one thing, the Greeks had introduced an almost fatal division between the head and the hands. Thinking, an ennobling exercise, could, in fact should, stand above, beyond, and apart from operations. This separation was for long, and to some extent still is, a source of mischief both in the way we seek to educate and in the way we try to conduct our operations. Then too, in the extending search for further knowledge, men did not for a long time find much of the kind of information that would help to simplify the day's work. Without much apparent interest in such direct application, they lacked also the instruments and methods that would produce evidence appropriate for such a purpose. So in the tilling of the fields, the transport of goods, and the construction of homes and public buildings, things went along about as they always had.

Somewhere near the end of the sixteenth century, things began to change. Many causes and many minds contributed to this gradual shift in intellectual affairs. Such names as Copernicus, Galileo, Kepler, Gilbert, and Harvey suggest the general nature of this developing alteration. More precise definition of what was happening can be found in some phrases pulled from the texts written by two other remarkable men. In his notebooks, Leonardo da Vinci wrote, "Whoever appeals to authority applies not his intellect, but his memory—Those sciences are vain and full of errors which are not born of experience—and which do not terminate in observation, that is whose origin, middle or end, does not come through the five senses—this is the rule to be followed by the investigators of natural phenomena; while nature begins from causes and ends in experience, we must follow a contrary procedure, that is, begin from experience and with that discover the causes."

Francis Bacon, a more contentious spirit, brushed aside

the "delicate learning" which held "that the dignity of the human mind is impaired with long and close intercourse with experiments and particulars." He, like Leonardo, argued for investigations, "subject to sense and bound to matter." And he went a good deal beyond his fellows in explaining the purpose of such investigations. The object was, by learning, to establish "dominion over natural things" so one could act "to relieve and benefit the condition of men." It is parenthetically interesting that three hundred years later a man defined for a group of electrical engineers in Philadelphia the point of their profession in almost precisely these same words.

In summary, men at work by the end of the sixteenth century were beginning to supply the pursuit of knowledge with earthier methods and more mundane aims than had marked the pursuit theretofore. The concern turned more and more from speculation and received opinion to careful observation and from the search as ennobling exercise to the search for useful evidence. The result of all these labors produced, not surprisingly, a considerable disturbance both in the intellectual world and in the world of affairs. Throughout the seventeenth century, there were tedious and painful efforts to connect one freshly discovered thing with another and to supply general propositions that would, it was said, save the new-found data. Along the way, as the recently acquired information began to displace older assumptions or explanations taken on faith, there were painful and dislocating debates over the structure of the universe, the nature of reality, and the meaning of existence. The life of the mind, oscillating in these years between polar differences—the ideal and the useful, things unseen and things subject to the senses—was vivid, exciting, and at times very confusing. But within the confusions it is possible to determine some dominating tendencies. The track of most of these tendencies lies through the larger history of ideas and outside the present purpose.

But one of the tendencies is to the point here. In the *Novum Organum,* in 1620, Francis Bacon gave his fullest statement of the need to search for that practical knowledge which could be applied to relieve and benefit the condition of men. From there, a gathering momentum under increasing control passes through such points as Watts's condenser, Faraday's dynamo, and Maxwell's equations and on to the computerized machinery that put men on the moon.

It is the hope that some feeling for the nature of that momentum—the push of ideas—and some sense of the increasing control—the tightening connections between new evidence, evolving ideas, and subsequent action—may be derived from the following pages. As men in this country moved from the perplexities of a small canal lock in the wilderness to mastery over electrical systems of great sophistication and power, they were carried along by this accelerating process.

The energy in the momentum derived from many sources: hard, indeed in this day, almost unimaginable, physical labor; the intuitive perceptions of countless builders; the weight of accumulating experience. But the prime source was the play of intellectual forces. Constantly refining methods of investigation, men steadily increased their knowledge and understanding of the world around them and then applied what they had learned to modify the stern conditions of that world. And by taking all this thought, men have come almost to the fulfillment today of the Socratic objective; they know enough to enter the company of the gods and to sit with them in authority.

This point achieved, it now turns out that knowledge is only one part of power. The other part is an understanding of how to use it, and in this area men still fall somewhat short of the divine comprehension. As suggested at the outset, men now know a great deal about nature and about the parts of the technology they have created to take the place of many natural things. But they are without the sense of a general purpose for the organization of the parts, a scheme that would enable them to introduce a saving order among the pieces. As a precondition for the development of such a scheme, it was also suggested at the outset, men must accept themselves—the fact of human being, warts and all—as the controlling factor in the design problem.

This is not to say that the search for a ruling concept should be made only among the uncertainties of the human affections or the whimsicalities of human being; that the power of reason which brought such great advances in the past three centuries should now be shoved aside. For one thing, the technology that now surrounds men, that must be taken into account in the development of any general scheme, was created by and responds to the exercise of rational processes. Therefore, any satisfying program for modern man in his technological universe, while it may be sustained by an act of faith, must be fashioned by acts of the intelligence.

For another thing: It is true men have affections; it is true they are often whimsical; but it is also true that they think. Indeed, that is, perhaps, their distinguishing characteristic. The concern for the qualitative does not necessarily drive out the quantifiable. The scheme of values that seeks to give appropriate room for the feelings cannot seek, as is sometimes believed, to protect those feelings by the exclusion of the cerebral cortex.

All this was put with his usual clarity and force by Alfred N. Whitehead. The business of "philosophers, students and practical men today," he said, was "to recreate and reenact a vision of the world." It should contain elements of the radical and conservative, of the reverent and the orderly, a vision "penetrated through and through with unflinching rationality." "There is now," he concluded, "no other choice before us; either we must succeed in providing a rational co-ordination of impulses and thoughts, or for centuries civilization will sink into a mere welter of minor excitements."

Such is the main line of argument of this book. Much of its weight lies at the far end of the narrative. That narrative begins with those Americans who did not know how to run a level or build a lock but were determined to construct canals as the first support for what they called the "stupendous" vision of "a new American age." Starting from that point in the wilderness, the line runs directly to the present necessity to reenact some even larger vision for the world.

CHAPTER 2

Building Things
in Early America

THE TOWN of Peterborough, New Hampshire, was incorporated in the year 1760. At that time about 280 men, women, and children lived within the township. Almost all of them were settled on farms where they grew their own food; made their own boots; spun, wove, cut, and stitched their own clothes; and confected their own medicines. In the town, there was a water-powered saw and grist mill and one store. One road, wide enough to hold a yoke of oxen, ran twelve miles south to New Ipswich. Trails for a man on foot or a horse and rider took wandering courses east and west to connect the town with other small settlements in the region. Not many travelers made their arduous way along these paths, nor had they much cause to do so. "We must think of Peterborough" at this time, says the town's historian, "as a collection of more or less isolated subsistence farms."

Sometime in the decade following the incorporation of the

town, the house I now live in was built by a man named William McNee. It stands today in all its essentials, save heat and light and plumbing, almost exactly in the state of its original construction. The cellar is thirty-five feet long by twenty-seven feet wide by six feet high. The cellar walls are made of fieldstone laid up dry. In the center of the cellar is the foundation of the chimney. It is twelve feet square; also of fieldstone, also laid up dry. The chimney rising from this foundation is built of sand-struck brick and is large enough to serve three fireplaces and a Dutch oven. The house is framed with six by six hewn pine beams pinned together with mortise joints. Within the frame, on the ground floor, are four rooms. The ceilings of these rooms are constructed of horsehair plaster, while the walls are, in the kitchen, made of pine boards, and in the other rooms of half plaster with a base of pine-board wainscoting. Over each fireplace, covering the chimney breast, is feather-edge clear pine paneling. Upstairs is an attic enclosed by the roof of rough finished rafters, pine boards, and shingles.

Not everything in this structure is on center, trued up, or worked out within precise and uniform dimensions. What is now the living room is two inches wider at one end than at the other. In the room where I am now writing the wainscoting runs around three of the four walls. The height of each wainscot differs from that of the other two. No doorway in the house is similar, in height or width, to any of the other seven. On the west end of the house, looking out to the mountain from the second floor, is a window that seems to be centered on the ridgepole. It is actually five inches off the center.

Such irregularities appear throughout the structure. They are probably the result of starting somewhere and figuring out the next step as one goes along, of trusting to the eye, of letting the board nearest to hand determine subsequent width and heights. The result is a casual asymmetry in detail that is considerably more satisfying than exactitude. And the whole represents a masterful distribution and organization of interior space. Moreover—from the pitch of the roof and the height of the ceilings and the shape of the back fires to the disposition of the windows and the width of the foundation walls—form follows function.

William McNee built his house, as his neighbors did, with his own hands, assisted no doubt by those neighbors when the frame was raised. Clearly, as he began, he had a general scheme in mind. A look at other houses built about the same time and still standing in the region indicates how much one is like another. That scheme was the early New England farmhouse, called by real estate agents today a Cape Cod Cottage or simply a Cape.

This farmhouse, like the ship of the line of the eighteenth century or the DC-3 of forty years ago, represents one of those moments in man's building history when the essential factors in construction—available materials, the level of individual competence, aesthetic judgment, and intended purpose—were brought into satisfying combination and given almost perfect expression. Not many structural solutions developed in this country have exceeded the New England farmhouse either in art or in common sense. Working within this scheme William McNee, uneducated, untrained, a farmer in a wilderness, fulfilled its sternest requirements. The house he built has stood, a small monument to a remarkable conception, for over two hundred years.

Soon after this dwelling was finished, a good number of William McNee's neighbors built houses for themselves. And in the next twenty years there were many more neighbors and many more houses. By 1790 the population of Peterborough had increased fourfold. What happened in that town happened all over southern New England. Throughout the

region from the Connecticut River to the Atlantic Ocean
there were to be found a steadily growing number of thriving
communities in the ten years after the Revolution.

It soon became obvious that roads wide enough for a yoke
of oxen and forest trails for men on foot were insufficient
means for the kind of transport such an expanding territory
required. It then further became apparent that any network
of roads to tie the various parts of the region together would
take a great deal of time to build, cost a considerable amount
of money, and present continuing difficulty in the maintenance. So a search was made for a reasonable alternative. As
men in expanding communities had done for three thousand
years, the southern New Englanders turned, in time, to the
idea of using the existing watercourses.

From Boston, which had become the intellectual and financial center of energy for the region, there came a plan to
connect rivers by short canals to create an extended transpor-
tation system. The thought was to use the Charles and Concord rivers from Boston to Lowell, where a connection
would be made with the Merrimack. From that junction the
line would extend north through Manchester and Concord to
the town of Franklin in the center of New Hampshire. At
that point, the line would turn west and proceed through a
patchwork of brooks, small lakes, and canals to the town of
Windsor on the Connecticut. As a further elaboration, the
passage could then be continued down that great river to
Long Island Sound, then west along the sound to the Hudson, then up the Hudson to Albany, and then, by a means
not fully worked out, west through New York State to Lake
Ontario and, from there, to the mouth of the St. Lawrence.

Such were the dreams in some men's heads in 1790 at a
time when not a single successful canal had been built in this
country. In the event, no more than a fragment of this general design was realized, but in that fragment one can find

most of what one needs to know about the origins of systematic engineering in this country.

The narrative begins in 1793, when the General Court of Massachusetts gave a group of private citizens the right to form the Middlesex Canal Company and build a canal between the Charles and Merrimack rivers from Boston to Lowell, a distance of about twenty-six miles. These men asked Laommi Baldwin to take direction of the job. He was a sometime cabinetmaker, an occasional surveyor of boundaries, a citizen of Woburn designated in the town records as "a man of learning." This distinguishing citation arose, no doubt, from the fact that he and his friend Benjamin Thompson, later Count Rumford, had walked from Woburn to Cambridge to attend the lectures of John Winthrop at Harvard on mathematics and physics. Together they had also contrived an apparatus to assist them in the performance of some experiments in the physical sciences.

When Baldwin was appointed superintendent of the works, the first thing he did in the spring of 1793 was to assemble the tools. Here is the essential inventory. For clearing and digging: axes, hoes, shovels, mattocks, crowbars, scythes, pitchforks. For working wood: saws, foreplanes, halving planes, draw shaves, chisels, holdfasts. For working metal: forges, vises, anvils, tongs, files, chisels, hammers. For working stone: drills, chisels, wedges, priming wires. The list included every important tool available in this country at the time and almost all the instruments men had used to build things for a thousand years.

The next step, in the summer of 1793, was to gather a work force—men known to be good at building stone walls or framing barns, handy men in the local towns, and most of all farmers, who, like William McNee twenty years before in New Hampshire, had learned how to build and repair whatever they needed for their work or their living. By the end of the summer, Baldwin had collected the best tools and the most skilled work force available in the United States to undertake the new venture. It was then discovered that men who had learned how to take care of themselves and who, working within a general architectural scheme, had left small timeless monuments without number to a remarkable conception, had neither the wherewithal nor the knowledge nor the skill to even begin to build a canal.

The place to begin was to run precise surveys and levels. This, in the opinion of Henry Knox, a resident of Boston, a hero of the Revolution, secretary of war, and a great supporter of the Middlesex Canal Company, was "more a matter of accurate perceptions and judgment than of science." Therefore, the thing to do was to look for a local man rather than for someone with experience from abroad. "Upon the morals and steadiness of our own people we may depend, while foreigners in so many instances are defective in these essentials." Acting on such advice, Mr. Baldwin asked his friend Samuel Thompson, a magistrate in Woburn who had done some surveying, to undertake the task. Using a compass, his eye, and such accurate judgment as he possessed, Mr. Thompson produced some disastrous calculations. It was later discovered that in the six-mile stretch between Chelmsford and Billerica he had made a vertical error of forty-one and a half feet. Baldwin then spent three days with a man named Cross building a leveling instrument out of "an iron screw, some loops, and four pieces of wood." After a week in making observations with this device, a committee, traveling by chaise "to carry victuals and baggage," concluded that it could not be made to serve the purpose. Thus, at the very outset Baldwin and his fellows confronted a problem—the taking of accurate levels—that was to puzzle and bedevil canal builders in this country for two decades.

In the course of that first year, they confronted other prob-

lems large and small that they found they did not know how
to solve. Most of them were posed by an element—water—
and a force—flowing water—they had never worked with.
Consider this list. They found they did not know how to ex-
cavate a ditch with expedition, that is, how to proceed
through rock, how to dig earth in quantity and dispose of it
in appropriate places. They found they did not know how to
seal the ditch effectively so that water would not run out
through the bottom and sides. How, as they said, to keep a
canal from weeping? They found they did not know how to
build retaining walls that would keep their form. They found
they did not know how to design a canal lock and what to
build it out of. Wood, brick, stone? They found that they
could not lay up either brick or stone with a mortar that
would retain its holding qualities under water. They found
they could not design the machinery for the opening and
closing of the valve gates for the locks and even if they could
design it there was no one in Massachusetts who could manufacture it. They found, in sum, they they did not know
anything about how to build a canal.

Their situation seemed proof of Henry Adams' sardonic
judgment delivered a hundred years later: that Americans
"struggling with the untamed continent in 1800 seemed
hardly more competent to their task than the beavers and
buffalo which had for countless generations made bridges
and roads of their own." Even at the time, John Stevens,
reflecting on the difficulties confronting the builders of the
Middlesex Canal, concluded "without further preface" that it
would be more sensible to invent something that did not
exist rather than to try to build another canal. He proposed,
two decades before there was a locomotive on this continent,
the construction of a railway with "innumerable ramifica-
tions" that could be used to transport goods more cheaply,
faster, and more safely "in every direction." The steam car-

riage, when it came into being, "would move against a fluid 800 times more rare than water, and thus would no doubt attain a speed of 100 miles an hour."

In spite of all the obvious discouraging prospects, the men of the Middlesex Canal persisted in their venture. Finding no American who knew more than they, they sensibly waived the requirements of morals and steadiness and looked to foreigners for help. In time two men were found. The first was John Rennie, a young, upright Englishman who had drained and reclaimed great tracts of marsh on the Solway Firth. He had also been active in the construction of harbors and docks at Wick, Torquay, Grimsby, and other coastal towns in the British Isles. Reluctant to interrupt his work at home, he gave advice by mail. For "cuts of fourteen feet or less" nothing was better than spades and wheelbarrows. As for embankments, "where earth is to be carried into a valley at a distance less than 30 yards—use wheelbarrows; 30–100 yards use man carts [large wheelbarrows pulled by a horse]; 100–400 yards, single horse carts."

Such counsel was no doubt useful, but Laommi Baldwin and his fellows needed advice more direct, specific, and continuous about their own job. Late in 1793, they heard that there was a man in Philadelphia named William Weston who might be persuaded to help them. He too was a young Englishman, and had come to this country to supervise the construction, just begun, of a short canal to join the Susquehanna and Schuylkill rivers. It was said that he had worked with the great James Brindley, who had built a canal for the Duke of Bridgewater, and it was known that he had built a bridge over the Trent and a turnpike near Gainsborough.

In the early spring of 1794, Mr. Baldwin took a two-week trip to Philadelphia to see if he could persuade Mr. Weston to help with the problems of the Middlesex Canal. The visit went well. Mrs. Weston expressed "a passionate desire" to

see Boston, which all Englishmen thought was the "most interesting" city in America, and besides Mr. Weston was for
the moment at liberty. The first thing he had done in Philadelphia was to rip out all the workings that had been done on
the canal site by local labor; then it was discovered that there
was no money to begin new construction. Mr. Weston was
soon to find that this kind of thing happened quite often in
early American engineering ventures. In any case, he said he
would come to look at the Middlesex Canal in the summer.

Before he did so he sent forward by coastal sloop a spade,
a wheelbarrow, and his own leveling instrument, a telescope
with an attached spirit level. This instrument was not much
help because, pending Mr. Weston's arrival, no one in Massachusetts knew how to use it, and the wheelbarrow, to Mr.
Baldwin's dismay, got lost in transit. "The Barrow," he
wrote to Mr. Weston, "did not come. Pray send the dimensions of one with a section figure in each direction with
length, breadth, and height, diameter of wheel, and whether
wood or iron, etc."

In July, Mr. Weston came to spend two weeks and in that
time he did wonders. To begin with, he used his leveling instrument—the first time such a device was used in this country, it is often claimed—to run accurate levels throughout the
entire course of the canal. Besides this, he advised Mr. Baldwin that wood was not as good as brick and brick was not as
good as stone for building locks. He also advised him not to
try to clear out and use existing watercourses but to build a
canal separate from and parallel to the brooks and rivers.
(The great Brindley had told a committee of Parliament that
the only reason God had made rivers was to feed water into
canals.) Mr. Weston then went on to say that to seal the
canal prism—or trough—one puddled. That is, one took a
clayey soil and poured water into it and then stirred it with a
heavy paddle until the mixture became a smooth-running

paste. Then one laminated the trough with layers of this paste until the trough was watertight. Sometimes the lamination reached a thickness of two feet. Mr. Weston also drew up some preliminary designs for locks and for the machinery for opening and shutting the valve gates of the locks. He further arranged to get the parts for this machinery cast in a foundry in New York from molds he himself made. Then he went back to Philadelphia. But for the next five or six years, he corresponded with Baldwin on problems of construction and design.

It is not beside the point here to say a little more about William Weston. He was one of those men, like Christian Senf of Sweden and Benjamin Latrobe of France, who came to this country in the seventeen-nineties because, as George Washington told John Randolph, "finding no competent workman here," those wishing to dig canals or build bridges "must invite a proper person from Europe." He was one of the best and most resourceful of these visitors. From his arrival at Philadelphia in 1793 to his departure in 1801, he did the following things: consulted on the building of the locks that joined Wood Creek with the Mohawk River at Rome, New York—the aborted first effort at the Erie Canal; prepared a plan for a water supply for the city of New York with an ingenious system of reservoirs and distribution centers; examined the Lancaster Turnpike and recommended a new kind of foundation and surfacing material; designed the piers for the Market Street Bridge in Philadelphia, sinking the foundations in cofferdams to an "unprecedented" forty-two feet below the surface of the water.

First and last, he had a hand in about every significant engineering project that was going forward in this country at the time. Knowing not much, he knew a great deal more than anyone else and was in frequent demand. Pursuing his lawful occasions around the country, he came high and lived at the same level. For his six weeks, including travel time, on the Middlesex Canal he was paid $2,107.60. For his brief look at the locks on the Potomac, he received $1,440.00. While making what were called his ocular surveys, he saw to it that he was well supported by goods and services. It is pleasant to reflect on his processions through the total wilderness of Virginia, Pennsylvania, or New York, followed by three or four of his clients, several axemen and rodmen, a devoted servant referred to in the manifests as his "MAN," and two or three horses laden with excellent meats, aged cheeses, and cases of Madeira. Traveling always with such substantial reinforcements for his person, he was also always generous of his time, advice, and supplies. For his clients, he made as full and complete reports as he knew how. He kept in touch with jobs after he had left for other ventures. He lent out not only his spade and wheelbarrow, but also his precious leveling instrument, to people who but dimly understood the level's uses, and he always saw to it that his MAN was well supplied with porter. He was withal a valuable and attractive force in our early engineering development and perhaps the exciting model for succeeding generations of well-rewarded consulting engineers.

It would be pleasing to report that after Weston's departure all went well with the construction of the Middlesex Canal. But such was not the case. Years of exasperating difficulty continued to try the patience and indeed the spirit of Laommi Baldwin and his fellows. Let us look at some of the difficulties. First, there were constant problems of excavation. It was very hard to cut through and extract the roots of trees in the wooded areas and much harder to cut through the sections of solid rock. Second, the structures, even those built to Mr. Weston's designs, frequently fell apart or washed away. For instance, Mr. Weston had said that stone was better than brick or wood for canal construction. So, for three years of hard labor men using stone worked on the first lock in the Merrimack River. On the day the work was completed the superintendent made this entry in his diary, "opened— the first lock. Broak and failed." The trouble was that the stonework underwater foundation had disintegrated. Third, in spite of the fact that Mr. Weston left behind his leveling instrument with instructions for its use, there was constant maddening trouble in running satisfactory levels, a trouble that continued in this country for twenty-five years wherever levels were run. Fourth, although the walls and bottom of the ditch were lined with puddling material, the canal continued, as men said, to weep. In fact, it always leaked.

The sources of these difficulties were many, varied, and interesting to consider. Some had to do with tools—or the lack of them. There were no stump pullers, no root cutters but axes, and no way to go through solid rock except with cold chisels. An engineering crew that had to send three hundred miles to a foreign expert to get the dimensions for a proper wheelbarrow was, not surprisingly, short on all kinds of necessary instrumentation.

Some of the difficulties had to do with materials. If it was hard to cut through rock with cold chisels, the work could be simplified by blowing the rock apart with powder charges. And this was done, but not with any very great success, because the explosive capacity of the charges was always severely limited. More significant was the limitation of the mortar. The reason the first lock "broak" was that the mortar had lost its holding qualities. What was needed was a hydraulic cement that would set up under water. The Romans had known about such cement—pozzuolana—and had used it almost two thousand years earlier around Florence. Following the collapse of the empire, the substance had dropped from general use. John Smeaton tried it out when he built the Eddystone Lighthouse in the middle of the eighteenth

century. He had read about it in a book by the Frenchman
Bernard de Bélidor, who had never worked with it himself
but had read about it in Vetruvius. By the time the Middlesex Canal was being built, therefore, hydraulic cement was
known about, but its properites were not well understood
and no one thought it could be found in America. The proprietors of the canal finally obtained a substitute—Dutch
Trass—from the island of St. Eustatius, but there was continuing trouble in mixing it in correct proportion with lime
and water.

More than tools, more than materials, men proved the
main source of difficulty in the work on the canal. Take the
question of leakage. Weston had explained that the way to
stop leaks was to puddle and he had described the very simple procedures for puddling: Laminate the walls with layers
of paste until a shield two feet thick is obtained. The thing
was to get the shield thick enough. The great Brindley had
given the ultimate prescription. Some men came to him as he
lay dying and asked him how to prevent weeping in the canal
they were building. "You puddle," he said. They said they
had. "Then," said he, "puddle again—and again—and
again." The men on the Middlesex Canal never quite followed the prescription. They took neither the time nor the
trouble to get a correct consistency in the puddling material
and they took neither the time nor the trouble to build the
layers of the material to a proper thickness. So the canal
always leaked.

And take the question of levels. When there is a proper instrument, the rest is just a matter of accurate readings and
simple arithmetic. After Mr. Weston's visit, there was
always a proper instrument at the Middlesex Canal—first his
and then one bought at Mr. Weston's suggestion from Mr.
Troughton in London. Yet there were continuous errors that
seem to have derived from two sources. First, the readings

made were not always precisely taken by the men; second, the instrument itself was often out of adjustment. It was a sensitive thing; in careless usage the cross hairs drifted out of alignment and the level moved off true. Those using the instrument banged it about and took neither the time nor the trouble to make the necessary adjustments. So small initial errors became compounded and grossly exaggerated as the running of the lines proceeded.

These are simply examples of the wayward and inept performances that spread through every part of the building of the canal. Looked at from one point of view, that building can be seen as a continual and almost systematic botching of a very simple process. From another point of view, it can be taken as an exercise rather more remarkable in its execution than that which put Neil Armstrong on the moon in about half the time.

The problem presented to Laommi Baldwin and his fellows was not, in some ways, unlike the problem presented to the queen when she was given straw and a spinning wheel and told to produce a roomful of gold. She knew about straw and she knew about spinning wheels, but she did not know from any previous experience how to put the two together to do work. And whatever work she might find out how to do was supposed to wind up with a specific but unusual end product. All this combination of novelty in causes and effects produced in the queen, as is well known, a devastating confusion over even the smallest detail of the project. It was the same in the canal. Take the case of that wheelbarrow and its proper dimensions. Of course Laommi Baldwin knew about wheelbarrows. The Chinese had used them in the later Han era and every farm around his home town of Woburn had one. But he was looking for a wheelbarrow that would do a new—even if a very simple—thing. He wanted an earth mover that, in very rough conditions, under continuous usage, could carry a maximum volume of dirt with a minimum expenditure of energy. Hence, the interest in the difference between wood and metal wheels and in a new design. And within limits, this need for adaptation and innovation held true for all the tools and materials the men used on the canal. To fit the conditions and purposes required by this new task, they all had to be modified in varying degrees.

As with materials and tools, so with work procedures and practices. Most members of the labor force came from the same background as William McNee. As farmers, they had proved nimble with hand tools; ingenious with stonework that was laid up dry; competent, at times gifted, at building with pine beams and boards shaped within normal tolerances of three or four inches in twenty feet. On the canal they were working for the first time in a collective venture where one man's labor affected the performance of all the others. They were putting together unfamiliar structures. Above everything else they were working with a strange force—flowing water—and they were seeking to contain and control that force within quite narrow and specific limits.

Nothing in their background prepared them for the exacting routines required in such an enterprise. To puddle with a care for the correct consistency and a concern for the nice application of each layer in the laminated whole and then to puddle again and again and again in the interests of making the good enough perfect—none of this was to be found in the sanctions under which they had previously labored.

As with materials and tools and procedures, so with nice calculations and sensitive instruments. The eye had served them well enough in dealing with ordinary problems of scale and proportion in their building and even in matters where exactitude had higher claims, as in surveying. Anyone who has read an old deed knows, for instance, that in running a boundary it was often taken as sufficient to cite a spot six paces east from the old oak tree that had been hit by lightning. In the regular work of the day, therefore, precise observation and measurement were new requirements, hard to come by, harder to believe in.

By the same token, there were very few sensitive devices—indeed devices of any kind other than hand tools—that were used in the performance of the day's work. Men who had spent their lives with hammers, saws, scythes, and pitchforks had trouble developing a feel for careful handling and precise adjustment. Indeed, for a long time they looked upon the telescope and level as something as "mysterious" as a magician's wand. It must also be remembered that there was in the atmosphere within which these men worked no supporting sense of what machines of any kind were like. For one thing, there were not many machines anywhere in the world at the time, and for another, the British had seen to it by legislation that their colonial possessions should not learn even what there was to know about machinery. Only two years before a start was made on the Middlesex Canal, Samuel Slater, working from his memory of the carders and water frames he had used in England, completed the first textile manufacturing establishment in this country at Pawtucket, Rhode Island. In that same year there was, almost certainly, only one operating steam engine in the entire nation. How, in such conditions, to think about a mechanical problem, how to get the feel of a mechanical context, how even to learn to use or care for any kind of machine—small and delicate or large and powerful—posed, indeed, a great difficulty for ordinary workers.

If little could be salvaged from their own previous experience to help the builders of the Middlesex Canal, even less that was useful could be discovered in any of the available literature. Laommi Baldwin, as a man of learning, had acquired some propositions dealing in a general way with the nature of the physical world. He had read the *Principia* and understood such enlightening equations as $F = ma$, but he could find no way to translate such generalized understanding into theorems that could be applied to the building of a canal. Nowhere, for instance, could he find formulae to help him calculate the volume of water flowing in a channel of known dimensions or to help him determine the most effective design and spacing arrangement for bridge or aqueduct supports. Beyond that there were no handbooks available to describe the simplest procedures—how to seal a canal prism, how to lay up a retaining wall. Baldwin and his fellows proceeded in their labors unsupported by any organized body of knowledge that could be related directly to what they were doing. It does almost seem that the buffalo and beavers of Henry Adams, guided only by primordial instinct, were better prepared for the task at hand.

Instinct, whether at work in beavers building dams or birds making nests, dictates not only ways and means, but the shape and structure of the end result. The men on the Middlesex Canal were, at the beginning, not only unsure of methods and materials; they were uncertain of what the characteristics of the finished product should be. Deprived as they were of programs designed by instinct or previous experience or adequate knowledge, they were in a position of peculiar difficulty. It is that which makes a study of their situation especially interesting.

In the painful, wasteful performance of their essentially very simple exercise, they demonstrate the fundamental nature of the connection between doing and knowing. Knowledge as it expands tends to extend the range and increase the variety of the dictates of instinct. Where the beaver sticks to his dams, men with growing understanding can proceed from canals to railroads to airplanes to rocketry. Knowledge expanding does another interesting thing: it can supplant the

prefigured conclusions of instinct—the design of a nest—
with reasonable predictions of the performance characteristics of a product yet to be built. For instance, when Donald
Douglas started to give concrete expression to his greatest
conception, he knew enough to know quite precisely what
the DC-3 could do when it was finished. The same was true
for the men starting out to design and build the interacting
system of rocketry for the moon shot. They knew enough
about ways, means, and the calculable potentials of things
never before produced to plot a sensible development and to
have confidence that the result predicted would become the
result achieved.

Such competence in the process and confidence in the end
as hoped for was not extended to the men on the Middlesex
Canal. They knew that what they were doing had been done
by others elsewhere and in more favoring circumstances.
They had the conviction that what they were doing was a
social, economic, and political necessity. They had common
sense, imagination, considerable experience in building other
kinds of things, intuitive judgment, and very impressive determination. But they did not know enough, and so they
were brought—as all others who had tried to do what they
were doing in this country before them had been brought—
to the point of utter failure.

What took them through this point of crisis and put them
on the other side was William Weston. On matters where
they were ill-served by their previous experience, by the
available literature, and by their own ingenuity, he supplied
the information that fortified all their other assets and capacities. He did not in fact know much, and some of what he
knew was inappropriate for the circumstances. But he knew
enough to give clearer shape to designs that could only be
imagined before his coming, fuller definition to practices,
and actual demonstration of principles that had not been suf-

ficiently revealed by earlier experience. He could also, almost
by his presence alone, explain to the men on the canal that
what they were doing was possible to do because it had been
done before and he had seen it done and had himself worked
with the man who had done it best.

That man was James Brindley, who had built the Duke of
Bridgewater's short canal. And in the building, he had
learned a great deal about the construction of canals, which
he had put into his magisterial aphorisms. Some of these
have been quoted in the preceding pages, and in the later literature there are many more references and appeals to his authority. The things he said, compiled in the memory of a
growing number of his followers, became an engineer's man-
ual. And those who followed him understood what they
owed to him.

Fifty years after Brindley died, thirty years after William
Weston had come to tell Laommi Baldwin what he had
learned from Brindley, James Geddes was the chief engineer
of the western division of the Erie Canal. One of his most
difficult problems was posed by the terrain around Rochester, New York. Here a series of abrupt changes in elevation
in the land through which the Irondequoit Creek flowed appeared to dictate the need for a rather elaborate system of
locks. Standing at the site one afternoon, he suddenly perceived, in a moment of "triumph," how this whole system of
locks could be supplanted by a single aqueduct.

Perhaps he had in his mind's eye as he was making his survey of the rugged terrain "the crowning triumph" of James
Brindley sixty years before. In building the Duke of Bridgewater's canal, Brindley had solved a somewhat similar problem by erecting his famous aqueduct—thirty-nine feet above
the surface of the water—over the Irwell River. At any rate,
at the moment of his perception, Geddes thought to himself
how delighted "the great Brindley with all his characteristic

anxiety to avoid lockage" would have been at the thought of this solution.

Brindley was, to all intents and purposes, illiterate. He did all his building without benefit of written calculations or drawings. What other men learned from him was acquired by work with him or by observation of his finished structures or by recollection of his earthy sayings. Such learning as was in him passed on by word of mouth. By such means, what Brindley found out about canal building near Manchester, England, in 1759 was moved across three thousand miles of ocean and six hundred miles of wilderness until sixty-five years later it reached a man at work on a canal near Rochester, New York.

That is the way knowledge about building things traveled in those days. Consider the nature of this communication loop a little further and in a little more detail. In 1793, William Weston was brought from England to advise those who wished to build a canal between the Susquehanna and Schuylkill rivers. Most of the advice he had to give came from what he had learned from the work of James Brindley. In 1794, Mr. Weston, in the course of an eight-week visit to Massachusetts, imparted this same advice to Laommi Baldwin, who was trying to build the Middlesex Canal. During the next six years, Mr. Baldwin followed this advice as well as he could with due regard for changes caused by limitations in available materials, money, and the skills of an untutored labor force. It cannot be said that by this process he evolved a new kind of American Practice. Given the adverse circumstances, he discovered a good deal more about what not to do than he learned about exactly what to do and exactly how to do it. But he did finish a canal that almost always worked almost well enough, and in so doing acquired an understanding that put him ahead of all his fellow canal builders in this country by the turn of the century. What he had learned from William Weston, as modified by his own experience on the job, he in turn communicated to his son Laommi. And in 1821 Laommi the younger was called to Pennsylvania to finish the canal between the Schuylkill and Susquehanna rivers that had been begun thirty years earlier by William Weston. In the event, Laommi the younger did not stay to complete this task. He became engaged in a great public quarrel with Samuel Mifflin, the president of the canal company, over the proper width for the canal. Laommi the younger had the support of the lore that had come down to him from Brindley to Weston to his father. He had also the support of canal measurements he had taken in Europe during a trip some years before. Mifflin relied upon the opinions of others and a misreading of a description of how a canal had been built in Ireland. But he had presidential authority and his views carried the day. A year of experience with the finished work demonstrated the error of Mifflin's design. So his installations were ripped out and the canal was rebuilt at great expense in accordance with the original plans as put forward by Laommi Baldwin the younger.

What happened in Pennsylvania and Massachusetts should suggest that what knowledge of engineering existed was held in the minds of a few widely separated men; that the network for the retention and distribution of the available information was an unstable coalition of personality and accident; and that the means for enlarging the body of knowledge were insufficient and randomly assembled. Earlier history goes to the same point. In the thirteenth century the Chinese had built the Grand Canal, connecting the Pei-Ho with the Yang-tse-Kiang. In the fifteenth century the Italians had constructed a network of small canals. In the seventeenth century the Canal du Midi was completed in France under the direction of Paul Piquet. This extraordinary waterway contained 119 locks in 148 miles and rose at one point to an elevation of 620 feet above sea level. But very little of what men learned in the course of these enterprises had been transferred to other places. When in 1759 James Brindley began his "ochilor servey or a ricconoitoring" for the Duke of Bridgewater's canal he went forward with procedures made up out of his own head because he had no real information about what had been done before.

Considering all this, it must be taken as a considerable demonstration of ingenuity and persistence that what Brindley then found out in England made its way sixty-five years later into the mind of James Geddes in upstate New York. Moreover, given these circumstances, what was planned as possible in this country in the years from 1790 to 1810 seems remarkable and what was actually achieved appears truly marvelous.

In spite of such favorable assessments, it must be obvious that the building of the structures required by an expanding society rested in that time upon extremely precarious foundations. The art painfully acquired in one small enterprise like the Santee Canal at the south, was rarely transferred to those at actual labor in some other small enterprise—like the clearing of Wood Creek in New York. What men learned in any one place and any one time moved slowly, if at all, into the consciousness of men working at later times in other places. There was no formal process by which one could expect with confidence to build a body of knowledge secure enough to sustain a developing profession.

Perhaps by 1800, the level of understanding and the strength of the communication network were sufficient to insure that an important piece of evidence—such as the uses of pozzuolana—would not drop out of sight and mind again for eighteen hundred years. But the slippages and wastes in the system for distributing information produced damaging inefficiencies. For instance, twenty years before William Weston

was brought to the Middlesex Canal with his leveling instrument and his, apparently, unique ability to use it, David
Rittenhouse had not only made but extensively used such instruments himself in Pennsylvania. No one in Massachusetts
knew this. For further instance, twenty years after men on
the Middlesex Canal had learned that it was not sensible to
build locks of wood, proprietors of a small canal three
hundred miles away in New York were trying with disastrous results to build wooden locks. For yet further instance,
twenty-five years after hydraulic cement had been brought
into Boston from St. Eustatius for the locks at Chelmsford,
men building locks around Rome, New York, had to redis-
cover the uses of such cement for themselves. Little bits of
hard-won knowledge, fragments of partial understanding
were strewn in disorder around the country at the sites of
small, often half-finished, projects.

What was obviously required at the turn of the century
was some large-scale, long-continuing engineering exercise
that would draw together existing information, stimulate the
search 'for further understanding, consolidate what was
known and what was found out into a sustaining body of
knowledge and that, above all, would offer to a large number
of men the opportunity for extended, systematic practice in
the uniform application of the knowledge that they learned as
they built.

Such a "stupendous venture" began in upstate New York
thirteen years after the Middlesex Canal was completed.
Along the 363 miles from Albany to Buffalo, men working
for eight years on the Erie Canal laid the secure foundations
of the engineering profession in this country. One of those
who acquired the fundamentals of his calling on this great
enterprise was John Bloomfield Jervis. What he learned during the construction of this watercourse through the wilder-

ness, what, in his subsequent career, he did as a builder of dams, bridges, aqueducts, locomotives, and railways—all this taken together makes the record of his life almost a history of American engineering in his time. Some of his remarkable achievements are the subject of the chapter that follows.

CHAPTER 3

The Works of
John B. Jervis

JOHN B. JERVIS, given his natural bents and persuasions, grew up at the right time and, more particularly, in the right place. He was put in the middle of one of the most favorable of those combinations of fate, character, and contingency that Charles Beard called the course of history. There was not much in his early surroundings to suggest such good fortune. At the time of his birth, December 14, 1795, the prospect was that in any man's lifetime things would remain about as they had in his father's, grandfather's, and great-grandfather's day—or as far back as one cared to go. And the place he came to live in when he was two years old appeared to hold a more solid position in the past than in the present. Fort Stanwix had been a revolutionary battlefield and had twice been the site of treaty agreements that deprived the Iroquois Indians of their birthright. But in 1797, renamed Rome, it was a small village set in the forests primeval of upstate New York. All his life John Jervis carried with him the sensation, stronger than memory, of the wild and isolating atmosphere of those endless woods.

Most of his boyhood was spent there working for his father, who was a farmer and lumberman. He learned early to sow and reap, to handle an axe, to drive a pair of horses in rough terrain, and to tend a sawmill. During occasional sessions at the common school he learned to read, write, and factor. At home he read the Bible, the *New England Primer*, and the *Institutes* of John Calvin, which he found "a sobering and substantial book." For the rest, he worked in field and forest from sunup to sundown and thus it continued until he was twenty-two.

There was no reason to believe that it would not continue that way all through the foreseeable future, as indeed it did for his father and most of his neighbors. But in the summer of 1817, Benjamin Wright asked John Jervis if he would help to cut a path sixty feet wide through a cedar swamp on the outskirts of Rome. Wright was a close friend of Timothy Jervis, John's father. He was a leading citizen in the village and chief judge in the local courts. He had also just been appointed superintendent of the middle section of the proposed Erie Canal. That section was to extend from Schenectady to Montezuma. Rome and the cedar swamp lay on the line of the canal about midway between the two communities.

For numberless years animals and men had made their way across upper New York State along a chain of waterways formed by the Mohawk River, Wood Creek, Oneida Lake, Oswego River, and a network of brooks and creeks that fed the Finger Lakes. For at least fifty years, men, recognizing a desirable end long before they possessed the necessary means, had discussed the possibility of a canal from Albany to Buffalo. The project recurringly appeared in campaign oratory, in debates in the legislature, in economic tracts, in newspaper descriptions of an inevitable imperial expansion, and in the talk of tavern customers. How the great dream and the arguments from political and economic necessity and all the idle chatter were reduced through the years to a practical program, soundly conceived financially and administratively, is in itself a remarkable story. But it must be left here with the summary statement that by 1816 a body of canal commissioners appointed by the state was ready to think seriously about the building of a canal 363 miles long across the width of the whole state.

They thought first of all of the difficulties and of how little they knew of the task at hand. And then they thought, as others had thought so often before them, of an obvious solution. They sought the services of William Weston and offered him $10,000 a year to take charge of the enterprise. But Weston had been back in England for fifteen years, he was getting on and he felt the claims of domestic felicity, so he refused. In such a pass, Joseph Ellicott, one of the commissioners, said, "It does not take a wizard or magician" to use a leveling instrument or lay out a canal, and he urged the appointment of a local man.

It may have been the most important remark that had been made in the history of American engineering. Consider what happened when the commissioners acted on it. They looked in upper New York State and found four "principal engineers" to undertake the supervision of the construction of the canal, James Geddes, Charles Broadhead, Benjamin Wright, and N. S. Roberts. Three of these men were judges and one was a schoolteacher. The judges had picked up the rudiments of surveying while running boundaries to settle disputes among their neighbors. Two of them, James Geddes and Benjamin Wright, had had some experience in the years before 1816 in making what might be called preparatory feasibility studies of various canal routes through the upstate territory. N. S. Roberts, the schoolteacher, taught himself simple surveying after Benjamin Wright had persuaded him in 1816 to take part in the venture.

In other words, at the start of this great enterprise the four men charged with the responsibility for its direction had no previous experience with canal construction, had little or no practice in building anything, and, so far as one can find, had never used a leveling instrument. The tools in their possession at the outset were those available to the men on the Middlesex Canal twenty years before. The labor force, as on that earlier occasion, was recruited from the farmers, laborers, and odd-job men who lived in the vicinity.

Starting with such assets in 1817, the men on the Erie Canal taught themselves how to do the work they had undertaken. Geddes and Wright, for instance, laid out a circle with a thirty-miles radius around Rome and practiced running levels on this line until their separate findings varied no more than an inch and a half in fifty miles. They then went on to learn how to design and construct locks, weirs, dams, reservoirs, and aqueducts. They learned how to puddle until the channel was sealed; they learned how to find, prepare, and use hydraulic cement. They learned how to build all kinds of new machines to break up matted turf, to move earth and rock, and, most of all, to cut roots and pull stumps. The stump puller was a marvelous contraption of thumbscrews, gears, and wires with wheels sixteen feet in diameter. And they learned how to organize and direct the labor of 4,000 men and 2,000 horses and oxen.

As in any learning, there was a good deal of waste motion, trial and error, time lost, and false starts. They had to find out on their own that wood was not a sensible material for locks. They continued for quite a time to have trouble with levels; they produced bad designs for weirs and reservoirs; they lost a good many poorly constructed foundations and retaining walls. In the first year they sent Canvass White abroad to make a careful study of European practice. He brought back rules and procedures that greatly advanced the understanding of the local builders, but it took a good deal of time to adapt what he had learned to American conditions and materials. What in the end the local builders relied on most was their own ingenuity and persistence.

After eight years by these means they completed what was called over and over again in those days this "stupendous" enterprise. As there had been a certain magnificence in the conception, there was a kind of grandeur in the execution. Never before in this country, save in the revolutionary armies, had so large a force of men been put together to achieve a common end. And these men, with little more to sustain them than muscle, native wit, and an organizing purpose—which many people thought an idle dream—built an ordered structure conceived from rational premises through 363 miles that were for the most part a trackless wilderness.

In so doing, they built a good deal more than a canal. For one thing, of course, they changed the history and condition of life throughout a considerable section of the new country. For another, they freed men who wanted to build and make things in this country from their dependence upon European advisors and European rules of thumb.

Finally, in constructing the canal, they opened the first— and quite possibly the best—school of general engineering in this country. Acting under the direction of the remarkable chief engineer, Benjamin Wright, scores of untutored men learned how to think and work their way through unfamiliar problems. From this experience these scores of men went out to build with ingenuity and confidence many different kinds of things in many different parts of the country. Taken all together, they were the principal agency in the accumulation, codification, and consolidation of the information that gave to our engineering its first sustaining body of knowledge. What they discovered on the Erie Canal was a feeling for materials, an understanding of simple mechanisms, an increased sense of and respect for certain natural forces, together with an increased sense of and respect for the kind of nice procedures that are necessary to contain and use those forces in an orderly way. Most of all, perhaps, they discovered a new set of attitudes: that it was possible, by taking care and thought, to devise novel means and methods for dealing with all kinds of problems both old and new; and that it was possible to think and act on a grand—indeed heroic—scale.

John Jervis was one of the first and certainly one of the most astute students to enter this school. He came with his axe to cut through the cedar swamp near Rome in the summer of 1817. His first lesson came on his first day. He was a very good man with an axe but he had never had to cut down trees along a line that had been precisely laid out and he had "a little trouble" for a time in conforming faithfully to the plotted requirement. It was a very small lesson, but he never forgot its larger implications. He began to learn, along with many others, that in building even simple structures respect for exact calculation must often supersede the suggestions of even the practiced eye.

As an axeman he worked often with the surveying party and, again along with many others before him, he found in their exercises "a profound mystery." But he observed with care and asked a good many questions. Slowly he began to understand the meaning of the various procedures, but by the end of the summer he felt he had "seen only a very small edge of the great field." The "mystery of the level, the taking of sights, its adjustments, and the computations of these observations were all dark to me." Seeking ways to penetrate the darkness, he asked Benjamin Wright at the end of the summer's work if he could begin the next spring as a target man. Wright agreed and suggested Day's *Principles of Navigation and Surveying* and Flint's *System of Geometry and Trigonometry* as winter reading. Early in 1818, Jervis started out in a party directed by N. S. Roberts to complete the survey of what became known as the Rome Haul. Roberts combined the temperament of a taskmaster with the instincts of a schoolteacher. He encouraged Jervis to make practice levels after work and to plot the line and profile of the canal on a map during rainy days. He took the time to review the young man's results and subject them to the severest analysis.

Thus a sort of pattern of instruction was set. For the next seven years Jervis passed through an orderly progression of titles and duties—axeman, target man, rodman, tally man, surveyor, resident engineer on a subdivision, superintendent of an operating division. At each stage he moved into a larger sphere of action and at each stage he had a solicitous superior to review his work—N. S. Roberts, David Bates, Canvass White. And always—at all stages during these years—there was Benjamin Wright on his biweekly supervisory trip, available for consultation, support, and suggestion. By such means, Jervis learned everything to do with the task at hand, from levels to stone work, from blasting to keeping accounts, from the design of aqueducts to the management of working parties. For one year he directed maintenance on a finished section of the canal, and found that maintenance with all its repetitions and regularities bored him. But since the canal was always leaking somewhere, and piers washed out, and mortar crumbled, and lock machinery broke down, he had a great deal to do and he learned a great deal. Especially he learned that one saved time, money, energy, and anguish if it was done right the first time.

This course of instruction was not without attendant hardships. Men worked twelve hours a day, seven days a week. They often walked in rough going, twenty miles a day. They worked in all kinds of wind, weather, and temperature. Occasionally they lived in farmhouses along the line, but more often in lean-tos or tents in the forests. For such exertions there was not, in terms of money, much reward. In his first year, Jervis received $12 a month and in his fourth year as a resident engineer he was paid $90 a month.

After seven years, the canal was finished and Jervis was ready to move on. The work on the Erie had produced an epidemic of what was called "canal fever" and there were opportunities for experienced men all over the country. Benjamin Wright, the source of all wisdom on canal building, became a sort of clearing-house for such opportunities. Everyone turned to him, including a group of men who wished to build a waterway from Carbondale, Pennsylvania, to New York City. Their object was to develop a cheap means to bring coal to Manhattan, which at the time was obtaining its fuel from England and Nova Scotia. Wright became the chief engineer for the project and appointed Jervis his principal assistant. Since Wright was acting as a consultant on six or seven other ventures, he gave his young associate a very free hand in both the planning and the execution of the work on the 105-mile canal.

In 1825, Jervis conducted his preliminary survey of the terrain on horseback. The proposed route ran for a considerable distance through the valley of the Delaware River. At one point Jervis found himself on a height of "rocks [that rose] nearly perpendicular two hundred feet above the river." He had from this eminence an exciting view of a long stretch of forbidding terrain. "The turbulent action of the water" far below, "the general gloom," heightened "by the swirl of a heavy snowstorm," and "the wild surrounding of the scene" made an impression on his mind "that fifty years have not eradicated." At the time he concluded that these were conditions "more severe" than he had ever dealt with, which "certainly presented a very unfavorable situation for a canal."

Jervis, because so much of his youth had been spent in the solitude of empty space, may well have been especially sensitive to the sight of wild landscapes. But such scenes were ineradicably impressed upon the minds of many of his closest associates in those days. And, as a colleague of mine, an engineer, wistfully remarked, "There was a kind of grandeur in this lonely, purposeful labor in the wilderness." It was usually in the wilderness that these men practiced their profession, and from their experiences they developed, not surprisingly, strong feelings about nature and their own work and the relationship between the two. Ten years after Jervis stood on the high banks of the Delaware, John Childe was making the first survey of a railroad across the Green Mountains into Pittsfield. Standing one afternoon on a promontory, he saw laid out before him a dramatic composition of sheer cliffs, roaring water, and tortuous valley. It was the kind of place where no man had ever thought of putting a locomotive before. Caught between awe and interest, he threw his cap in the air and cried out, "What a place for engineering!"

There is in that cry much of the spirit that informed the whole profession in those days. These young men went directly to surrounding nature to find their problems, and nature stated the case back to them within clearly fixed conditions, but fairly. Nature thus became part of an adversary process, but also, in an interesting way, an *amicus curiae*, a force to conquer which offered the terms by which conquest became possible. The result was an interchange, a symbiosis, that worked to the advantage of both parties. Jervis believed implicitly in this relationship. Years after his work on the

Delaware and Hudson Canal he built a railroad along the banks of the Hudson and came under fire from those who believed that this construction would scar the beauties of nature. In his brusque way, which grew brusquer as he got on, he replied that ugly erosion of the shore would be prevented by his neat embankments, that trees thus secured from undermining would grow more beautiful, and that "the railway thus combining works of art with those of nature would, in fact, improve the scenery." In this timeless collision "let those who would," call him "barbarian," and of course, a good many did. But nothing ever said deterred him from the faith that what he was doing improved not only the scenery but man's lot and also that what he was doing was an art.

He was a master of the precise fulfillment of all the requirements of proved procedures—puddling, grouting, running levels, digging foundations deep enough, and the like. He could design conventional structures—locks, bridges, dams, and aqueducts. He was at home with simple machines—stump pullers, gating systems—and had some familiarity with small steam engines. Just as important as this command of the fundamentals was his attitude toward the work. The Erie Canal had been an extended exercise, hard to come by in the more self-conscious and abstract forms of later engineering education, in the overriding necessity to improve the means. Jervis had learned never to look at any process without seeking a more satisfactory solution. This meant not only better ways, but more information.

Thus prepared, he started on the Delaware and Hudson Canal. In addition to his own assets, it is worth noticing that he had the help of others. Benjamin Wright made occasional visits and working with Jervis all the time were six men he had brought with him from the Erie Canal. Their presence created a sort of engineering seminar and was yet another demonstration of the continuing intellectual influence exerted by what men had learned in their time on that great enterprise.

Shortly after his first survey, Jervis decided (one hopes he had Brindley in mind) that he could save a good many locks by converting the last seventeen miles at the western end into a railroad. His plan was to traverse a very steep grade—at one point 900 feet above the river bed—by a system of eight connecting inclined planes. Great reels of cable, powered by stationary steam engines, would pull the coal cars along rails set into these inclined planes. For the final four miles of the road, where the grades were negligible, Jervis planned to use the power of steam locomotives.

At the time he put these ideas forward there was one short inclined plane railway in this country, and on the whole continent, there was not a single locomotive. The directors of the Delaware and Hudson, who had formed a company to build a canal, were, not surprisingly, somewhat resistant. But the arguments of Jervis and the persuasions of Wright produced in time at least their acquiescence.

To prepare himself, Jervis went to Quincy, Massachusetts, to see the inclined plane railway built there to take granite from the quarries. He saw nothing that would help him in his far larger enterprise. Then in two books he found pictures of the machinery used on the inclined planes built by the British for their coal-mining industry. He thought these machines were "too cumbersome to secure convenience of operation." So, out of his own head, he designed a very simple system of reels and sheaves. Thus he obtained the means to pull the cars up the steep grades, but he needed also a way to get them down the hills under controlled speed. He had no great confidence in the durability, under large loads, of the friction brakes that had been developed in Europe. So he conceived the idea that "atmosphere could be made to do this work." After a series of painstaking experiments and careful calculations, he created a "pneumatic convoy," a set of four wooden sails, twenty square feet in area, for each car. In the event, this convoy worked, but Jervis added friction brakes as an insurance measure.

The locomotive power for the last four miles of the railroad posed a problem more complex. There were no locomotives on this continent in 1828; indeed, there were very few anywhere in the world and none of these worked very well. Not until 1829 did George Stephenson introduce the forced draft and tubular boiler that made his Rocket a convincing demonstration that these machines could have a serious use. But again Jervis had read a book or two, had seen some pictures, and had studied the subject with such care as he could. He concluded that steam locomotives constituted "a power that could be used with economy."

From there he set about drawing up specifications for the kind of engine he believed he needed. Like everyone else at the time, he had no way of telling how much a locomotive would pull and he had no reliable formula to assist him. He made some calculations about the "tractive power"— measured by determining the point at which wheels ceased to adhere to the rail and began to slip—but he produced nothing to help him predict how a locomotive would perform. In the end he was able to state only three desired characteristics: the engines should develop a speed of five miles an hour; the chimney stack should be no more than ten feet tall; the total weight should not exceed five and a half tons. This last specification was the most important. He had built rails of hemlock that he figured could bear a load of one ton per wheel. At first he hoped he could put six wheels on the locomotive, but reflection made him think that such a machine would have trouble on curves. So he reduced the number of the wheels to four—each of which he decided would exert a weight of 2,600 pounds on the rail. That he thought was an acceptable solution.

He gave these specifications to Horatio Allen, who had worked with him on both the Erie and Delaware and Hudson canals. In the spring of 1828, Allen went to England to purchase locomotives that would fulfill these requirements. Allen was a gifted young man of twenty-six who became a well-known engineer. This was his first independent mission. While in England he ordered four locomotives, one to be built by George Stephenson and three to be built by Foster Rathrick and Company. The latter was a builder of stationary engines; the single locomotive the firm had constructed was a primitive exhibition model made twenty years earlier.

These four engines arrived in this country in 1829. For reasons still mysterious only one of the four was assembled and put in working order. This was the Stourbridge Lion built by Foster Rathrick. On August 8 and again on September 9, it was tried out at Honesdale, the western end of the Delaware and Hudson Canal. Horatio Allen was at the throttle. On both occasions the machine—weighing over eight tons—crushed the hemlock rails. It was then put in storage and never used again.

That the Stourbridge Lion was the first locomotive to run "on this continent" was cold comfort to John Jervis. In fact he was "in no spirit" to claim or assume any honor. "The commercial object" of his interesting idea "had been defeated" and he was "sorely disappointed." He was also annoyed for the rest of his life that neither Horatio Allen, his agent, nor Foster Rathrick had held to his original weight specifications.

Still and all when he cast up his accounts at the end of the job in 1830, he could find sufficient cause for satisfaction. He had built 105 miles of canal through very difficult terrain at very low cost. This demonstrated his capacity to do the conventional work well. Beyond that he had revealed an aptitude for sensible experiment. True, in designing the machinery for the inclined planes he had made one considerable miscalculation that had caused him to believe he could use water instead of steam power on one level. But this mistake had been caught in time by a friend of his at Columbia University who had a better command of mathematics. And the whole inclined plane system turned out to be an impressive success. The air convoy never became a model for other constructors, but it proved useful as well as ingenious on the Delaware and Hudson. The loss caused by the failure of the locomotives was something over $12,000, but that failure had been produced because others had not followed his instructions. And against this deficit entry was the positive gain that he had learned something more than his fellows about roadbeds, rails, and locomotives. All in all, he concluded on his departure that "rarely has any company been more faithfully served."

Others, apparently, reached the same conclusion. As he finished the job on the canal Stephen van Renssellaer, John Jacob Astor, and John Renwick, the man who had discovered Jervis' miscalculation in the figuring of the inclined planes, asked him to undertake the building of the Mohawk and Hudson Railroad from Albany to Schenectady. This was in 1830 and it may be said again that at that time no one in this country knew with confidence how to build a roadbed, what to use for ties and rails, or what weight a locomotive could pull. On many of these matters Jervis could proceed with some confidence because of his previous experience. If he had no way to tell how to establish the most satisfactory and efficient grades, he knew how to construct and drain a firm right of way. This he did using a mixture of small stone and gravel. For ties he used stone where the grade was excavated and timber where it was filled. The rails fixed to these ties were of wood with iron capping. The real trouble for Jervis began when, early in 1831, he put a locomotive on the trackage he had built. The engine, called the Robert Fulton, had been built in England by Stephenson. It was twelve feet long, weighed about eight tons, and had four wheels four feet in diameter. Jervis reported that when the engine "encountered a vertical inequality in the surface of the rails there was a vertical motion at the end of the frame"— which was his way of saying that it bounced. Far worse, on curves the locomotive tended to wear away the rails and to lose its traction.

In England, where it was usually easy to lay tracks in straight lines in soil of uniform consistency, the four-wheeled engine presented no difficulty. But in this country, the changing conditions of ground and grade, reflected in rough roadbeds and sharp curves, made the smooth passage of the four-wheelers virtually impossible. What was needed was a design for an engine that would not bounce, rattle, wear away rails, or lose its traction.

Jervis, it will be recalled, had foreseen the theoretical probability that locomotives would have trouble on curves when he was thinking of his railroad for the Delaware and Hudson. Now he was confronted by the practical demonstration of the fact. For almost a year Jervis spent most of his time searching for a solution. In his effort he was joined by his old associate Horatio Allen. Allen had gone to South Carolina to build a railroad and had encountered the same problem. So twice within the year the two men met for several weeks of discussion in Albany. They knew to begin with only that someone in England had built an eight-wheel locomotive—two four-wheel trucks at either end of the machine that swung independently of each other. They also knew the engine had been a failure. Jervis had seen a drawing of this engine in a book and had concluded that it was simply too complicated to work. Allen, however, liked the idea of two independent trucks, each bearing equal weight. He therefore proposed a plan that would provide such trucks, each one supporting a separate engine fed by a common boiler suspended between the trucks.

Jervis opposed this scheme. Too complicated, he said. It involved the "operation of two separate pieces of machinery doing the same work." Besides, all the movement along the supporting frames would jar the steam joints and fittings out of working order. He proposed instead a six-wheel locomotive. The main weight of the boiler and engine would be carried by the two rear driving wheels, while the lighter front end would rest secured by a kingpin on a forward truck of four small wheels that could swing freely.

To this proposal, Allen objected. Too simple. The presumed complications of his own idea could be overcome by good design. The two debated the relative merits of their opposing views for six months before deciding that the only way to resolve their differences was for each to build an engine to his own plan. On November 16, 1831, the West Point Foundry Association accepted a contract to build a locomotive steam engine, "the said engine to be constructed agreeably to a plan of the same furnished and explained by John B. Jervis, Engineer of the party of the second part."

The crucial part of the plan was, of course, the forward truck assembly. But a few other specifications give an interesting indication of the state of railroad building in this country at the time. The engine had two nine-inch cylinders with a sixteen-inch stroke. The front wheels were made out of wood with a wrought-iron flanged rim. The whole frame was "seasoned White Oak timber." Another specification indicates the careful attention to detail that marked everything John Jervis ever did: "On the front end of the boiler a proper fixture to be made to receive a glass tube for a steam and water gauge so arranged as to admit of taking out a broken glass and conveniently substituting a new one, three extra glasses properly prepared to be furnished with engine."

The locomotive was completed in 1832. Called the Experiment, it proved, as experiments often do, something less than satisfactory on its trials. It had great trouble making steam; Jervis had hoped he could make use of the then unconventional anthracite coal but he designed so shallow a firebox that the fire never got very hot. Nevertheless, the locomotive ran well enough to prove the great virtues of the four-wheel forward truck. So Jervis, in the winter of 1833, rebuilt the Robert Fulton to include this front assembly. He called the engine the John Bull; on its trials it moved "with perfect beauty" and Jervis felt he might be pardoned for saying that his first ride on it was "a great delight."

It should be added that Allen's more complicated solution never worked very well and that the Jervis scheme became standard American design for a long time. In fact, in four years of discussion, experiment, and expensive trial he had solved what had become the major problem in American engine building and use.

The railroad interests recognized the great contribution John Jervis had made and offered without patent to their development and, on the whole, expressed a suitable gratitude by offering him in later years free passage on their right-of-ways. But there was a notable exception, which Jervis with his attention to detail duly noticed. "Mr. Vanderbilt does not know me, and though I daily see on his trains the truck and other devices I have invented and put in successful operation, he refuses me such compliment—. The railway fare that I pay is of no great importance, but I think I am entitled to the compliment, and as I see his trains pass I instinctively feel that I am not justly dealt with."

Soon after the John Bull was put in service in 1833 the work on the Mohawk and Hudson was finished and John Jervis went off to other things. During his eight years' experience with engines, rails, and cars he had developed feelings about the railroad that never left him. It was a new idea that was as important as the invention of the alphabet; an agency of revolution in the affairs of men, a moral revolution changing the diffusion of knowledge, the interaction of social relations, the prospects for peace, the extension of commerce and concepts of property. Then there was the locomotive itself. Nothing save nature stirred him as deeply. It was a perpetual source of "wonder and admiration." That such an engine "may travel in daylight, in the darkness of midnight, in sunshine and in storm, through cultivated fields and dense forests, through hill and over dale at the rate of fifty miles an hour, carrying hundreds of people as it thunders its way onward to the distant station and, in all its marvelous speed and power, holds fast to the narrow track, is truly a wonder; and though a thousand times witnessed, I never fail to admire and enjoy, as it passes with its long train, this splendid specimen of art."

Such feelings did not distort his recognition that the art as it developed in this country fell somewhat short of true fidelity to the highest canons. For instance, in designing locomotives little thought was given to the subject of size in relation to the work to be done. The rule was to make them as large as possible to pull loads, light or heavy, without regard to expense. The same with cars—"the prevalent idea" seems to have been "that a large coach gives importance to a railway whatever the dictates of cost, use and mechanical principles." As for rails, they were inferior, wearing away rapidly or breaking outright; as for roadbeds, they were insufficiently ballasted and badly drained. Little attention was given to the railway crossings, which created points of danger across the whole countryside. Stations, oversized and ill-placed, stood as monuments to something other than the convenience of passengers. In England, from fundamental engineering to satisfying appearance, the thing was better done. Here it was all a matter of getting quick results, cutting first costs, and creating imposing first impressions.

In this bill of particulars can be read much of the spirit Jervis brought to his own activity and much, as well, of the nature of American engineering at the time. He laid most of the disparity between American work and that of the Europeans to the operations of "UNFAITHFUL MANAGEMENT," which too often proceeded without regard to the claims of either stockholding "widows and orphans" or sound engineering principles. But all this, as used to be said, is getting ahead of our story and will be dealt with at greater length later.

Here the story must return to certain things Jervis did after he left the Mohawk and Hudson. At the time of his departure he had become, at the age of thirty-eight, one of the most experienced and well-known American engineers. He was therefore sought out by many varied interests that in the then rapidly expanding economy required many different kinds of goods and services. It would be instructive, and also interesting, to follow his career at length and in detail because he was for almost forty more years active in a series of changing ventures. But the purpose at hand will be served by a briefer, more selective process.

From the Mohawk and Hudson, Jervis returned to his earlier concerns as the chief engineer of the ninety-eight-mile Chenango Canal in New York. There was a special problem here. The surrounding rivers were unable to furnish enough water to keep a satisfactory water level in the summit section at all times. It was necessary to build a system of reservoirs to catch the run-off from the rains. The question was, what proportion of the annual rainfall would become available from the run-off? Both the size and the placing of the reservoirs depended upon the answer to this question. Jervis obtained from Europe a figure of 30 percent for this proportion. Having no good reason to doubt a rule that had been used for some time elsewhere, he nevertheless sought to validate the borrowed finding before building his reservoirs. Using an ingenious arrangement of sluices and rain gauges he discovered that the actual proportion of usable run-off was in fact 40 percent. Thus prepared, he laid out his catchment area and once again moved on to other things. He also duly noted some time later that his new figure had become the accepted "standard" everywhere.

Not long after this, in 1836, he was called to advise the commissioners on changes to be made in the Erie Canal. Some of these changes were required by the fact that the initial installations were wearing out, some by the fact that improved practice in canal construction had been developed since 1825, and some by the fact that heavy and increasing traffic had overloaded the original lockage arrangements. Jervis, after a careful examination of the whole system, proposed a new procedure for rebuilding the canal walls. He wished to introduce a more solid arrangement of backing stone, with closed-joint covering. He also proposed a new and larger lock chamber with dimensions based upon a formula he developed that expressed what he took to be the correct ratio between the area of the channel and the area of the canal boat.

The commissioners, to his disgust, rejected his plan for building solid back walls and spent a good deal more money on the facings than he believed necessary. They also, in disregard of his formula, built larger lock chambers than he recommended. In so doing they were moved, he believed, by a set of extraneous considerations since, he said, "they analyze nothing" that has to do with mechanics. Knowing that the canal was a big thing and an expensive thing, they thought it should be made to look big and expensive. "Superfluous cost was, in fact, considered a merit." As for size, the commissioners, pushing aside any thought of sensible ratios, accepted the idea that the largest possible hull without regard to the dimension of the channel was "the acme of economy." They had made no more scientific analysis of the situation than the simple-minded boatmen on the canal.

Shortly he was removed from such irritating distractions by the opportunity to do the greatest work of his life. This opportunity was offered in the fall of 1836 when the Commissioners of Public Works of New York City asked him to undertake the construction of a new water supply for the city. Water had presented a continuing municipal problem from the days in the last decade of the previous century when Aaron Burr had brought water into Manhattan through a system of hollowed-out logs. It will be recalled that William Weston had prepared a plan for the distribution of water throughout the city in 1798. The scheme had proved too ambitious for the resources of the time, and for the next forty years New York was served by a patchwork system that produced water unreliable in quality and insufficient in quantity.

By 1830, the city was expanding very rapidly, and it became obvious that some large-scale, carefully organized solution was necessary. The commissioners had turned for help to David Bates Douglass, a gifted man with considerable experience in the survey of boundaries and the building of military fortifications. At the time he was a professor of natural philosophy at the University of the City of New York. In the years 1834–1836 he conducted a thorough study of the whole problem, selected the Croton watershed as opposed to several other sources in Westchester County, ran the main lines for the aqueduct that was to transport the water from Croton to Manhattan, and drew up tentative plans for the supplementary structures that were to make up the whole system. Then he got into a bitter struggle with the commissioners over some ill-defined issues and was either pushed or fell from their good graces.

Opinions differ concerning Douglass as a man. Depending on the angle of vision he was found pure in heart, noble-minded, rigid, or cantankerous. It seems probable he was a mixture of all four (he was later forced from the presidency of Kenyon College by trustees who expressed their "confidence" in him and their "appreciation of his merits"). He was also, as professors of natural philosophy and its modern equivalents often are, something of an innocent in the conduct of human affairs. The cause of his departure, it appears, was a continuing collision between himself and the chairman of the Board of Commissioners, which was a reflection of their mutual confusion over the proper relationship between engineering and politics. Such a relationship, it may be added, is not simple to establish at any time, as others have discovered before and since. The problem was no doubt intensified by the conditions of that particular time. All parties to this great public enterprise were very uncertain, and therefore very nervous, over the question of whether or not the thing could be done at all. As Jervis said, "No experience in this country or hardly in modern times prepared anyone" for the construction of the Croton Aqueduct.

Yet he began work in October 1836 with his usual confidence and his usual care. Douglass had left a plan which in its general propositions met with Jervis' entire approval. As far back as 1825 he had, simply as a matter of interesting speculation, decided that the best source of water for New York was the Croton watershed. He approved also of the main line for the aqueduct that Douglass had laid out from the Croton River to New York City. What lay before him as he began his work was refining plans for the several major installations, settling details of all the structures, specifying as to kind and character of the work and forms of contracts.

The principal parts of the system were a dam and reservoir on the Croton River, a free-standing aqueduct running the thirty-three miles from the reservoir to the north bank of the Harlem River, a bridge over the river, and a set of pumping stations and distribution centers in the northern part of the city. The aqueduct itself offered Jervis the smallest difficulties in an engineering sense. In his days on the canals he had designed and built many smaller ones. The task was simply to repeat a familiar pattern over a longer line—thirty-three miles—while retaining a constant grade of thirteen and a quarter inches a mile. He had also to arrange a pattern for construction, and here again he was on familiar ground. Using the scheme he learned on the Erie Canal, he broke the whole line into sections four tenths of a mile long and let out each section to a separate contractor. Each section had a resident engineer; each group of five sections had a resident inspector of masonry. Every two weeks Jervis, his principal assistant, Horatio Allen, and the commissioners visited and inspected each section. In the building of this imposing installation one difficulty arose at the very beginning. Douglass had proposed to lay up all the backing in lime and the facing of the structure in hydraulic cement. Jervis insisted on hydraulic cement throughout. He therefore had an extended argument with the commissioners, who preferred lime because it was much cheaper. Only when Jervis said in a heated session that he would accept no further responsibility for the structure if lime was used was the issue resolved in his favor.

With a second great difficulty he had less luck. He had

designed a bridge fifty feet high to carry the water pipes across the Harlem River. Opponents immediately came forward to say that so low a structure would interfere with river traffic; that so low a bridge demonstrated that Jervis was not as bold as his predecessor Douglass; that what was needed was an "ornament," a "work of art that would be a credit to the city." To all of which Jervis replied that there was no traffic on the Harlem River, that unnecessary size was not a measurement of boldness, ornamentation, or art; that his design conformed to engineering needs and saved the city and state a great deal of money. The argument went on while Jervis stood firm. So, in his support, did the commissioners. The City Council refused to take sides. In this deadlock the opponents obtained from the state legislature an act specifying that at the Harlem Bridge "the underside of the arches at the crown should be not less than 100 feet above high water." Jervis, perforce, was left to design a bridge to these specifications and to speculate—which he gladly did—on a society that would save money by using lime in fundamental construction and spend money to obtain a pointless exaggeration of a proper function.

The major problem, in terms of engineering, lay in the dam and reservoir. To produce the head necessary to secure an orderly flow along the aqueduct grade the dam had to rise more than forty feet above the river. Since the river was about five hundred feet wide, the dam in both its length and height would have to be an imposing structure. And there were further complications. The Croton River, draining a large watershed, swelled dramatically during heavy rains and brought wild streams of water flooding through the valley. Finally, Jervis' survey indicated that while three quarters of the riverbed was solid rock the remaining one fourth on the north side was simply sand and gravel. A secondary but significant problem was posed by the fact that the water in the dam, falling forty feet, would act to erode the area around the apron of the dam at its foot.

Given these conditions, Jervis proceeded to build the dam in the following way. It was to have a masonry face backed by earth fill. The structure would rest, for three quarters of the river width, on the rock of the riverbed. The remaining one fourth would rest on wood pile foundations driven to refusal in the sandy bottom of the river. This was the first time that such piling had been used in a significant structure in this country, and neither Jervis nor Horatio Allen, in charge of the construction, was exactly sure how much weight each set of piles could bear. To break the fall of the water, Jervis put a reverse curve into the spillway of the dam, and to break up the flow of the water further, he put a series of timber cribs filled with loose stone at random through the flow off the apron at the bottom of the dam. A final feature should be noticed. The dam itself did not extend the whole way across the river. Anchored securely to the south bank, it was tied into the north bank by a retaining wall or earth embankment.

Because the whole system of installations was novel, because the construction took place in full view of the public, and because the departure of Douglass attracted considerable attention, the work on the aqueduct produced continuous notice and discussion in the newspapers and elsewhere. Not all of the attention paid to the project as it went forward was favorable. An Englishman named Borren sent a letter to the governor of New York saying that by his calculations the aqueduct would deliver "very little water." A professor of natural philosophy gave his opinion in a public lecture at Columbia that the Croton works as a whole were ill-designed and that, especially, the piping was "inadequate to the strain imposed." Then Douglass, in a letter to the commissioners, reported that by his observations things were moving toward "disaster" and indicated that he would be willing to do what he could "to correct errors."

All this fully exposed and argued out in public halls and in the newspapers had its effect upon the commissioners. They were charged with the responsibility, they felt, for a "stupendous thing," a "Herculean task" that seemed, if many presumably trained observers were to be believed, to be beyond the power of men—or at least of the men assigned to do this particular labor.

One morning Samuel Stevens, the chairman of the Board of Commissioners, came into Jervis' office. After some "casual conversation," he remarked "with a significant sigh" that it would be "sad if, after spending so much money, the aqueduct should be a failure." Jervis agreed but said he had no doubts; his "experience and investigation" gave (him) confidence in success. Since Stevens "could not be expected to follow the scientific reasoning—he must have faith."

This satisfied Stevens, but the fact was that the scientific reasoning used by Jervis required considerable fortification by faith also. In the matter of the pilings for the dam foundation, he had proceeded into an unknown area, and more significant, in the matter of the capacity of the aqueduct, he had entered a territory of great confusion. He had tried very hard to find some way to make a precise calculation of the volume of the flow and had discovered no sure way to do so. In fact, at the time no proved method existed. After considerable research, he had turned up three provisional formulae, one by an Englishman, one by a German, and one by a Frenchman. From these he had worked out a complicated compromise of his own upon which he based his design. Fortunately, when water was put into the structure the flow proved to be 25 percent more than his calculated amount, and fortunately, too, in every other characteristic the entire system, when finished, performed up to or beyond the designed specifications. By his combination of scientific reasoning and faith he had achieved a triumph.

But before that final triumph, he had lived through the greatest disaster of his professional career. By January 1841, most of the work at the Croton reservoir had been finished. What remained was to put the finishing touches on the earth embankment that tied the dam to the north bank of the river. The preceding December had been a month of constant storms, heavy rains, and heavy snowfalls followed by severe thaws. The river rose steadily until in the first week of the new year it reached an unprecedented height. A few inches from the top of the incomplete embankment, it found in the unfrozen earth a small passage. What soon followed is best described in a letter sent to Jervis by Edward French, the resident engineer. "I am sorry to inform you that the water about 3 o'clock this morning—in a few minutes swept the whole embankment and protection wall away. The masonry of the dam alone is standing—the line of the aqueduct has stood well. Every building below the dam that was not at least 25 feet above the river is swept away. Not a vestige of the wine works, or any of its buildings left and still worse, three lives lost. All bridges gone—."

There was, of course, a great hue and cry—much argument, many calls for scalps, feverish efforts to assign appropriate blame among commissioners, engineers, contractors, and an angry God. In the end it was decided that the only sensible thing to do was to rebuild the structure in accordance with lessons learned. During the angry debates Jervis had been urged to consider a way to put the responsibility on the Board of Commissioners. He did not do so. In summary of this whole sad event he said, "It was manifest I had been in error in regard to the extent of waterway necessary for so great a flood." He then, with the support of the commissioners, proceeded to enlarge the spillway of the dam and build a new retaining wall. A year later Edward French wrote him again. "As the people in the neighborhood of the dam say, 'the Croton today is mad.' " Rains and melting snow had produced another flood but, he concluded, "All is well." And so it continued.

The Croton Aqueduct was put into full service in 1842. Like the Erie Canal, it was taken both by those who watched its construction and by those who worked on it as an extraordinary achievement—stupendous, Herculean, one of the wonders of the world. In specifying the nature of the rock to be used in the building it was said "it is important that the aqueduct should last not only for ages, but for centuries." That was the mood of the men who put the work together. Since unlike the Erie Canal, which was for the most part a track through the wilderness, the aqueduct cut through a metropolitan area, many people came to share this mood. That structure became a forty-mile monument to what engineering could do for a society. It also became, again like the Erie Canal, a six-year engineering school. For a generation after, many of the dams, bridges, and railroads built in this country were designed by graduates of this school.

From this great venture Jervis returned to the building of railroads. Starting in 1847 with a short line along the Hudson River he moved, as did the industry itself, steadily westward. First there was the Michigan Southern and then the Chicago and Rock Island and finally the Pittsburgh, Fort Wayne, and Chicago, later know as the Nickel Plate. All three of these roads presented fairly simple and familiar problems; all three were at various times in precarious financial situations; all three were, Jervis believed, badly managed at the beginning and were built to standards somewhat below decent professional requirements. By 1864 he had gone about as far in his field as he wanted to go. At the age of sixty-nine he returned to Rome, organized the Merchants Iron Mill, and settled down to twenty years of peaceful life. During that period he did some consulting, kept abreast of developments in engineering by frequent attendance at meetings, and reflected continuously upon the meaning of his profession and its contribution to the life of American society.

Later in these pages an effort will be made to give some further description of the state of engineering in this country during Jervis' lifetime. Here, in conclusion, it may be interesting to take some brief further notice of Jervis as an engineer. It will be well to begin with some of his own summarizing reflections.

In the field, "you don't sit under an umbrella with folded hands" or "let notions of dignity prevent you from helping people." In other words, to get the feel of the job you may have to get your hands dirty. As for larger considerations, "A true engineer, first of all, considers his duties as a trust and directs his whole energies to discharge the trust with all the solemnity of a judge on the bench. He is so immersed in his profession that he has no occasion to seek other sources of amusement, and is therefore always at his post. He has no ambition to be rich, and therefore eschews all commissions that blind the eyes and impair fidelity to his trust." Since the profession was of the greatest importance to the public interest every engineering obligation must be taken as a public duty to be discharged with "scrupulous fidelity."

These are the words of a man in orders. And indeed in all he did and said there is the sense of a spare and austere spirit in the service of some superior commitment. It does not seem, for instance, that until he left the field at seventy he ever took a vacation. Once he spent a month in Europe and looked at bridges and right-of-ways the whole time. Nor does it seem that he permitted himself many of the ordinary personal exchanges and indulgences. In the large collection of letters and papers he left behind, the subject matter, even in letters to relatives, is almost always canals and railways. The messages to and from his wife are on the whole laconic reports. Once she was moved to say she hoped "we will learn not to place our hopes and expectations on *bridges*"; and once she said, "We both felt as if we wanted a quiet home of our own—but perhaps 'tis best we do not enjoy one."

Such scrupulous fidelity to the calling as all this evidence suggests was the source of the most obvious characteristic of Jervis' work. Given the available materials, the existing practices, the offered financial resources, he built as solidly as he knew how. His structures were complete expressions of his own integrity. This is, of course, the first and great commandment for any engineer, and many engineers have lived useful lives in single-minded obedience to it. But Jervis went beyond this essential commitment in several important ways. He moved always toward simplicity. If the British machinery for inclined planes seemed cumbersome, he designed less elaborate machines. If Horatio Allen proposed an eight-wheel locomotive tied together with too ingenious connections, Jervis came forward with his "too simple" four-wheel forward truck, which became "the first and most radical and universally approved advance in locomotive design."

As the speeches of senators, the symphonies of Shostakovich, and the poetry of the Pre-Raphaelites indicate, there is a tendency to inflate the expression when substance is wanting. This can happen as well in engineering as in any other endeavor, as the satiric constructions of Dr. Seuss suggest. At least as common, if more respectable, is the tendency to deal with the unfamiliar by creating the complicated. Allen's locomotive design is a good example. Many other examples could be cited from the history of men trying to come to terms during the last century with the novel force of steam. Some of the arrangements of boilers, cylinders, shaftings, and propellers that were put together to solve the problem of steam propulsion at sea make Dr. Seuss appear a careful student of nice design. It is a curious thing that fuller understanding of a complicated problem produces, apparently, an interest in finding a simpler way out—a search for what engineers call elegance. In engineering, as elsewhere, the principles of simplicity can no doubt be acquired through instruction; teaching ways to act successfully on this principle turns out to be difficult, indeed perhaps impossible. The need to search can be inculcated; the ways to find appear beyond the reach of formal pedagogy or even of experience. Jervis had within himself the sense of how to find the simple solution, which is probably one reason why he so often called the work he was doing an art.

But he understood it was not the kind of art that could go unfortified by increased understanding. At a time when most of his contemporaries were continuing to use painfully acquired rules of thumb, he strove always to enlarge his field of information in the hope he could improve upon the common practice. Confronted by his first locomotive, he searched for a way to calculate the tractive force; redesigning a canal prism, he looked for a formula; constructing the first artificial reservoirs in this country to serve a summit level canal, he obtained the evidence to modify a constant that had controlled all earlier practice. Such enterprise put him ahead of the beaver and the buffalo and also ahead of most of his fellows, who were relying upon customary procedures to work their way through the thickets of ignorance that surrounded engineering projects in those days.

Such enterprise also put him in a position of constant jeopardy. Moving always toward simplicity, acquiring information that enlarged his sense of the possible, he was, often, doing things that had not been done before. There was a price to pay—the Stourbridge Lion moved, in all, something less than two hundred yards; the air convoy proved to be merely ingenious; the Experiment never made enough steam to do work; the retaining wall at Croton gave way. But such costs demonstrate not only the degrees of difficulty in engineering at the time, but the boldness that was a fundamental energy in the spare, careful, austere spirit John Jervis brought to his work. His confidence, even before practical demonstration, in what his intuitive sense for simpler design and his powers of simplified reasoning told him, was the product of what he called his faith and what some others thought of as his overweening self-assurance. In fact, it was a marvelously controlled daring, putting him constantly in a condition of acceptable risk and putting him also at the head of his profession.

It suggests more about the profession than about himself that after he was fifty he discovered that while he was, as before, constantly moving from job to job, he was in fact merely repeating procedures now thoroughly familiar. At sixty-five, in search of something he had not done before, he started a small iron works. His instinct was, as usual, sound. If the places he had spent his life—canals, dams, bridges, railroads—were the main part of American engineering in the first half of the last century, the iron trade was another important part. But his connection with that trade, late in life, was more symbolic than real. To understand what was happening in that part of the profession, one can more profitably turn elsewhere—to such a man as John Fritz of Pennsylvania.

CHAPTER 4

John Fritz and the Three High Rail Mill

IRON WAS MADE in this country in the early years of the last century in the following way. Ore, in the form of iron oxide, was dug by hand out of the ground. This ore was put together with charcoal and heated. In this process carbon in the charcoal joined with oxygen in the ore to form carbon dioxide. The carbon dioxide, a gas, passed off into the air. In this way the ore was freed of oxygen. What was left was pig iron, a hard metal with a low melting point. It could thus be poured easily into many different shapes and castings. But pig iron fractured under stress because of the carbon in it. The charcoal that had freed the ore of oxygen had also in the course of the process added carbon to the ore. The way to get rid of this carbon was to heat the pig iron in a refining fire and then hit it with a hammer on an anvil. It was necessary to heat it and hit it a good many times to accomplish the desired purpose. What came from this process was wrought iron—a low carbon, malleable metal with many uses.

Henry Adams suggests that iron had been made this way since the days of Tubal-Cain, the first "instructor of every artificer in brass and iron." Tubal-Cain was the grandson of Methuselah and the half-brother of Noah. There is some truth in this suggestion, but it does not give an adequate impression of the shape and size of the industry as it was developing in the first decades of the nineteenth century. In 1830, for instance, about two hundred thousand tons of pig iron were produced in the United States. Most of this tonnage was made in iron plantations in the Northeast. The center of a plantation was the blast furnace. This furnace was, in effect, a ten-foot cylinder in a housing of masonry thirty feet tall and twenty feet square at the base. This cylinder was filled with iron ore, charcoal, and limestone. Workmen carried these materials in baskets across a bridge that ran from a hill or mound to the top of the furnace. At the bottom of the furnace was an opening through which air was pumped by a small water wheel to give a draft or blast to the fire. As the fire made its way up the cylindrical furnace, the ore melted and ran down to the bottom of the structure, where it was drawn off as pig iron.

To serve this central element in the plantation there was a considerable system of men, horses, oxen, and things. The most important things were available ore, woodland for charcoal, and running water for power. All this suggests a rural tract of sufficient size to insure a continuing supply of charcoal. In fact, these plantations were often eight to ten thousand acres of land set in isolated surroundings.

On this land lived sixty to seventy men and as many horses or oxen. What developed in such circumstances was a small community, self-contained from owner to common laborer, that has seemed to some feudal in its character and to others a counterpart to the plantations that lay to the south. The average annual production of pig iron for a plantation was somewhere around a thousand tons. This pig iron was sent out to small smithies and forges around the Northeast, where the metal was worked into wrought or bar iron and refined further into appropriate shapes for specific purposes.

That was the process in its classic form in this country in 1830. But in that year there were already things in train that would shortly produce a profound transformation in the iron trade. Some of these things had to do with new materials— coke, for instance, as a substitute for charcoal. Some had to do with ways to increase the intensity and influence of heat at every stage of the process—more powerful blasts of air in the furnace, more subtle ways of retaining and organizing the flow of the heat generated in the process itself. Some had to do with the development of new machinery to work the metal in both its molten and its solid form. The simple pounding of heated bars of pig iron to produce wrought iron, for example, was shortly to give way to puddling—or stir- ring—in a reverberatory furnace. And the work of eliminat- ing the carbon was further simplified by passing the puddled substance through mechanical squeezers. And finally the labor of shaping and finishing the bars of wrought iron by hand was greatly expedited by the creation of rolling mills. In these places the iron bars were passed through notched rollers that cut the material into desired shapes.

The sources of the transformation were many and varied. Some were borrowed from abroad, some developed in the years from 1830 to 1860 in America. The interaction of these sources and the varying rates of change in different areas are still matters of great interest and some dispute to students of the times. But all agree that about 1830 things began to hap- pen in the iron trade. It was also about this time that John Fritz arrived upon the scene to take some part in and, more significant, to give some direction to the transforming process. As just suggested, causality in this period of change is not fully understood, but it does not seem a matter of mere dramatic convenience to suggest that the foundations of John Fritz's career were laid in some part by John Jervis and Laommi Baldwin the younger.

It will be recalled that both these men had worked in canals that served parts of eastern Pennsylvania. The Delaware and Hudson had been built in the years from 1825 to 1828 to carry coal from Lackawanna County to New York City. Up to that time New York had brought most of its fuel from such distant places as Nova Scotia and England. The canal released it from such dependences; at the same time the canal opened great new opportunities for the coal trade in eastern Pennsylvania. Throughout that region there were extensive beds of anthracite, but little had been done to exploit them up to 1825. For one thing the seams appeared usually in rugged terrain somewhat removed from easy river transport. For another, anthracite was a new kind of fuel to most people, hard to ignite and keep burning.

The Delaware and Hudson put this coal within easy reach of many people, and these people, in a short time, became familiar with the characteristics and uses of this new fuel. So the demand and the production grew rapidly. Both were greatly increased by the finishing of the Schuylkill and Susquehanna Canal, which gave access both to new markets and to new coal fields in the southeast part of the state.

The purpose of the early mining was to find a new source for domestic fuel, but through the twenties an increasing number of blacksmiths and iron workers discovered that anthracite was a cheap and effective coal to use in converting pig iron into wrought iron and in working wrought iron into various shapes. They also found it could be used to serve the steam engines that were slowly taking the place of the old water powers. In short, in an industry that depended at almost every stage of its developing process upon heat, it was recognized in eastern Pennsylvania by 1830 that anthracite coal was a prime source of heat.

One of the sections of the state that was served by the Schuylkill and Susquehanna Canal was Chester County. This county, containing both ore and coal, was in 1830 a center for the developing iron trade. Here, on his father's farm, John Fritz was born on August 21, 1822.

It was, he recalled, a "well-regulated farm," where he worked all his early years. He learned how to drive a team and to plow and harrow. He also learned how to cut standing grass and grain by hand, using either a sickle or a scythe. Rising at four each day, going to bed not much after sundown each evening, he found his life and labor determined largely by the cycles of nature, which, fortunately, he loved. From time to time he went to a school, where he acquired only "the simplest possible things—reading, writing, and arithmetic." He was, for instance, told how "to properly hold a quill pen" and imitate letters drawn out by the teacher, but he was "never called on to compose a sentence or write an essay."

There was another, more important, distraction from the farm work. His father had a mechanical turn, and was in demand as a repairer of wheels and machines in the nearby flour and textile mills. John went with him on some of these trips and loved to sit among the works and watch his father taking things apart or putting them together. These occasional excursions and careful observations gave him the information he needed to decide what he wanted to do with himself. At the age of sixteen he was apprenticed to a blacksmith who had a shop in nearby Parkesburg.

Here he learned the trades of farriery and "country machine work." The tasks were the shoeing of horses, the ironing of wagon and cart wheels, the repair of farm machinery, and the making of iron parts for the grist and saw mills and small forges in the neighborhood. In the shop there were four smith's fires, four anvils, a set of taps and dies for cutting screws, a small iron lathe, a makeshift drill press, and some rolls for bending boiler plates. All these tools were of "crude character," but the instrumentation was more sophisticated and complete than could be found elsewhere in the district. The power in the shop came from a steam engine the smith had built himself. He had made his own rough drawings, prepared the forgings of each separate part, constructed the boiler, and fitted the whole together "without tools except makeshift."

The year Fritz entered his apprenticeship there were, so the Congress reported, 1,859 other stationary steam engines in the entire country. He was lucky to begin in a place where he could work so closely and continuously with this still unfamiliar new source of energy. Fifty years later he reflected that in all probability not one mechanic in a thousand could then build such an engine by himself. "Today," he said in 1890, "as many men work on a machine as there are parts of it. Present shop practice is better calculated to make machines out of men than to make good all-around mechanics."

Four years in the blacksmith shop gave him considerable experience in all kinds of simple metalworking. It also gave him, by chance, an opportunity to learn a good deal about engines. Living with the blacksmith was an Englishman who was the superintendent of the shops of the Philadelphia and Columbia Railroad. He occasionally asked Fritz to help with the repair of the locomotives, and often in the evening the two talked about "how machines ran." Parkesburg was about as good an elementary school in the mechanical arts as the society could supply in those days.

Fritz came away from this early schooling in 1842 with the

decision to enter the iron trade and a determination to learn
every part of the developing industry. As a beginning he entered that part which at the time was in the most unstable
equilibrium—puddling and rolling.

It will be recalled that the traditional way to remove carbon from pig iron was to heat the iron and beat it with hammers. Puddling was a simpler, faster way to accomplish the
same purpose. It took place in a reverberatory furnace that
was like a box inside a box. Here pig iron was melted down
by the heat from a fire that was separated from the iron by
the interior partitions of the furnace. The metal in a molten
state was then stirred or puddled by heavy wands or rods in-
serted through ports in the furnace wall. At the end of this
process the metal was drawn off, squeezed under pressure,
and became wrought or bar iron.

Rolling was the process by which this iron was given different kinds of shape, each shape uniform within its own
kind. The bars as they came from the reverberatory furnace
were pássed through pairs of notched or grooved rolls that,
by repeated passes through notches of descending size, cut
the bars to the desired dimension.

Puddling depended upon the availability of appropriate
ores, the successful control of heat, and the art of the pud-
dler. Rolling depended upon well-designed and solidly constructed machinery. At the time Fritz entered these processes, men in the iron trade did not know enough about the
chemical properties of ore, the influence of heat, the nature
of heavy machinery, or the canons of the art to proceed with
regulated means toward uniform ends.

Fritz was introduced to the difficulties of these developing
processes when he persuaded two Quakers, "the Messers
Moore and Hooven," to take him on as a common laborer in
a mill they were building at Norristown, not far from his
birthplace. The mill was one of the first in eastern Pennsyl-

vania to include both puddling and rolling; it was a kind of first tentative step toward the integration of an industry that had for a long time been divided among small furnaces, forges, and blacksmith shops.

The first job Fritz had was as a helper to the men who were assembling the machinery—rollers, boilers, squeezers, and furnaces in the mill. All these things were built on the job. Within a few weeks he was made a "regular mechanic," and within a year, when the mill was finished and he was twenty-two years old, he was put in charge of all the machinery. That meant maintenance, and from that maintenance he learned "his first great lesson." Power was distributed throughout the mill by a system of gears and cogs. As designed, it was like Horatio Allen's locomotive, an elaborate system which, in its elaboration, was forever "breaking up or getting out of mesh or creating a jam." In his first year in charge of this machinery he worked "day and night" taking out gears, cogs, and other moving parts. He had to do this work of redesign and reconstruction with hammers and chisels—"really the only tools"—and an instinct for simplicity. At the end of that year he had the conviction that if he ever built a rolling mill there "would not be a cog wheel in it," and he had a set of machines that worked fairly well.

At least the machines worked well enough so he could spare some time to learn by observation the puddling process, which he believed was the "most important part" of the whole operation because the production of good metal depended upon it. He spent every evening with the puddlers, watched them at work, talked with them continually, and finally decided that the reverberatory furnace had been very badly designed. After these observations, reinforced by his experience with gears and cogs, he concluded that all the major difficulties in the mill were caused by forms that were ill-fitted to their functions. He therefore went over every single part of every machine and piece of equipment in the mill seeking to make each one "work out better." In this constant study he had the assistance of members of the labor force, many of them English or Welsh workers who had, like the early steam engines and locomotives, been imported as indispensable parts of our industrial development. At first these men had viewed Fritz with suspicion, as a hostile agent in search of trade secrets, an unsympathetic student of tribal rites. But, recalling his days as a blacksmith's apprentice, he helped them move the bars around the rollers with heavy tongs and gradually won their confidence. So he heard from them over their pipes about the "manufacture of all kinds of merchant bar iron—flats, squares, rounds, boiler plates, tank plates, skelp plate for welded pipe, cut nails and spikes."

Things other than patience and curiosity apparently stood him in good stead. One day Mr. Moore asked him if he would take charge of the night shift—twelve hours—in the whole mill. Fritz was surprised and suggested several others who had been longer in the trade as more appropriate. "John," said Mr. Moore, "if I were going to look for thee in the evening until ten o'clock, I would come to the mill."

Fritz then accepted the appointment and later assumed direction of the day shift. He thus acquired an understanding of the entire process of puddling and rolling as it then existed. And he found, as others did, that in spite of every human effort, inappropriate ores (no one knew what made iron "cold short"—or brittle), uncertain control of heat, and breakdowns in machinery made the trade a precarious enterprise. Against such obstacles he labored day and night to make Norristown "the best plant" in the country, and by 1849 he "believed that [he] was doing it." But there were still other things to learn and so in that year he left to go to Safe Harbor, fifty miles away on the Susquehanna.

What attracted him there were two things: the building of

a rolling mill where he could put into practice all he had learned; and the building of an attached blast furnace which he knew nothing about. Safe Harbor was therefore a next step in his education and it was also a demonstration of the next step in the integration of the industry—the slow putting together of all the elements, from smelting through all the stages of refining and finishing. With a crew of Pennsylvania Dutch boys just off the farm, he built the plant from the ground up. Moving the heavy parts of the machinery and equipment by hand and putting them together with "two-handed chisels and sledges," they assembled the entire plant—mill and blast furnace—in about a year. And for another year Fritz remained to superintend the constant changes and improvements in the performance of the various parts. At the end of that time he was called away to start on the most interesting part of his life.

His journey took him out of the small anthracite furnaces, forges, and rolling mills in the eastern part of the state, across the Alleghenies, into the western regions of Pennsylvania. It was in this area that the foundations of the new iron trade—which later became "big steel"—were being put down by adventurous owners and manufacturers. The principal elements in this development were the substitution of coke for charcoal in the blast furnace, the increasing public demand for a single iron product—rails—and the integration of the manufacturing process from ore or pig iron through to finished product in a single system. When John Fritz came to Johnstown in 1855 as superintendent of the works of Wood, Morrell and Company, he began to take a directing part in what were in fact revolutionary developments.

What had happened at Johnstown in the five years before his coming suggests the precarious base from which these revolutionary operations were mounted. In 1850, the Pennsylvania Railroad was brought to the small city. At that time there were four charcoal blast furnaces in the area. In 1852 some Boston men, using money borrowed in Philadelphia, bought these furnaces and set out to convert them to the use of coke. Before the conversion was completed the Boston men discovered that they could not meet their obligations. So the Philadelphia creditors asked a man named Daniel Morrell, who knew little of the iron trade, to investigate the situation and propose a solution. What he proposed was a further investment by the men in Philadelphia. New money was again forthcoming but once again it ran out in 1855, before the new works was completed. Morrell knew little of ironmaking but he was resourceful and knew a good thing when he saw it. With these assets he persuaded a new group of men in Philadelphia to lease the ironworks for seven years. Thus Wood, Morrell and Company—usually known as the Cambria Iron Company—was formed to make rails out of pig iron made in coke blast furnaces. This history is typical of the development of most companies in the iron trade during the two decades from 1840 to 1860, when money was in short supply, the whole economy was in a state of fluctuation, and the nature of the trade itself was never fully understood.

At thirty-three, Fritz arrived in Johnstown, "a perfectly dreadful place" with streets of clay and sidewalks of wooden plank. Cows, dogs, and pigs mixed with the citizens on the principal thoroughfares. At the plant, on the outskirts of the settlement, he found an unfinished rail mill and three unfinished blast furnaces. The single furnace that worked was producing from local ores a pig iron that, to Fritz's now practiced eye, seemed "very inferior." In such unpromising surroundings, Fritz found his golden opportunity.

First, he finished all the elements—blast furnaces, reverberatory furnaces, squeezers, and rolling mills—that made the plant an integrated system for the production of rails.

Then he went into production and verified what he had predicted, that the pig iron from local ores was "very inferior." The bar iron made from it, when passed through the rollers of the rail mill, bent, broke up, or sheared off. What he needed was a new rail pile, a mix of various irons. The difficulty here was that no one could tell by simple analysis of the composition of the various irons what would make a good rail pile. As Fritz said, that "Queen of Sciences"— chemistry—was not then sufficiently advanced to permit such calculations. So he had to proceed by faith and experience to mix "cold short," "hot short," and what he hoped would be a good "neutral." The trouble was that the good "neutral" he found lay at some distance from Johnstown and was expensive, and these circumstances vexed the owners. There was a good deal of argument, as there always is when financial considerations are opposed by no stronger evidence than that supplied by faith. Finally matters were settled in the way Fritz wished. He obtained the neutral iron and produced a good rail.

But he still could not produce even good rails in quantity. As they passed through the rollers, they still quite often broke up or sheared off. The result was that the mill from the moment it entered production began to lose money. Worse still, as Fritz tried to push larger numbers of rails through the existing structure, the machinery became overloaded and so broke down. Time was lost and therefore money. And worse still, the overloaded machinery broke down in dangerous ways. Men were burned by molten metal when a ladle slipped its moorings; not once but twice a thirty-foot flywheel on a steam engine pulled off its axle and flew across the mill. Things could not go on this way. And besides, in the panic year of 1857 it was obvious that the owners could not go on this way.

Fritz was in the mill day and night during this period, observing every part of the process in the hope of finding some saving solution beyond the not very satisfactory measure of pushing men and machines beyond their capacities. One of the things he observed had to do with the point at which the rails were breaking up in the mill. The way these rails were made was as follows: Bars of iron, twenty feet long, heated to color, were laid on a table and then pushed through a set of two rollers. These rollers were notched and as the bars passed through the notches they were cut, in cross section, into the shape of the rail. Having passed through these notches, the bars landed on a table on the other side of the rollers. Here they were picked up by men with heavy tongs, brought back again to the table on the other side, and pushed through smaller-sized notches in the rollers. This process was repeated through successively smaller notches until the bars were cut to actual rail size. Fritz noticed that the rails tended to break up or shear off much more often on later passes than on the first one. It occurred to him that this must be because of the cooling of the bars as they were carried back from the receiving table to begin each time a new pass through the rollers. It further occurred to him that this cooling interval could be eliminated by adding on top of the existing set of rollers another set through which the bars could be passed and shaped on their return trip. He designed such a system—called the three high rail mill—in which the tables at each end could be raised or lowered to assist in passing the bars through the added rollers. It is interesting to notice here that a hundred years before Christopher Polhem, a Swedish engineer, had thought of the possibility of a three high rolling mill and one year before, in 1856, such a mill had been installed in a plant in Motala, Sweden. No one in this country knew of these Swedish developments.

The trouble with the Fritz design was that nobody liked it.

The men in the rolling mill had never seen anything like it and so opposed it totally. Ironmakers in the area told Daniel Morrell it was "a wild experiment," an idea of the "crack-brained Fritz that would ruin everybody." Fritz's old employer from Norristown, James Hooven, made a trip to Johnstown to say that if the three high mill was tried and failed his "reputation was ruined for life." The owners opposed it because it would cost a great deal of money. They saw no reason to put everything they had into a system for making rails that everybody said was crack-brained in a panic year.

Fritz countered with the argument that the mill as it existed would not make money in any kind of year and that he would have to have the three high mill or go elsewhere. In such a pass the principal owner came to the Cambria yards one Sunday morning. He and Fritz sat "on a pile of discarded rails with evidences of failure on every side." They talked over the dismal past, the difficulties of the present, and the uncertainties of the future. Fritz knew he had reached "a critical epoch." At last Mr. Townsend said to "go ahead and make your three high rail mill."

On July 3, 1857, the Cambria plant shut down while the new machinery was built by hand and in place. Twenty-six days later the job was done. Up to that time all rolling mills had been built with "breaking pieces" at dangerous points. The idea was that under unusual stress the supplementary moving parts would give way, thus saving the rollers themselves. Since in the mills of the time there were always places of unusual stress, the machinery was always breaking down, much to Fritz's irritation and at a loss of time and money. So he built this new mill as solidly as possible with no breaking points. His plant manager was much upset and argued for safety breakage points at spindles, couplings, and boxes.

No, said Fritz. "I would rather have a grand old smash-up once in a while than be constantly annoyed." "By God," said the plant manager, "you'll get it."

In the early morning of July 29, some of the owners, some of John Fritz's friends in the iron trade, and John Fritz met in the mill house to try out the new three high rail mill. "Conditions of secrecy had been imposed," to prevent the presence of the mill hands, who had set their faces and hearts against the change. Fritz and his friends heated a bar and passed it through the rollers. It worked. "You can judge," said Fritz, "what my feelings were as I looked upon that perfect and first rail ever made on a three high rail mill."

Shortly all rails in this country were made on the three high rail mill. It became the foundation for the developing industry. And for the next three years, as the great ironmaster Frank Jones later said, Cambria was "the cradle in which the great improvements which revolutionized the rail mills were rocked." Had he not been there, Fritz later believed, Cambria would have ceased to exist.

By 1860, the cradle was rocking in a very satisfactory but predictable way. Fritz was ready to go. After "six years of as hard, laborious, faithful, vexatious work as ever fell to the lot of man to do, I decided to leave the scene of my early struggles and try my fortunes elsewhere."

CHAPTER 5

The State of
the Art in 1860

IT cannot be supposed that the whole history of American engineering in the period from 1800 to 1860 can be extracted from the careers of John B. Jervis and John Fritz. The cast of characters is too large for one thing, and the fields of action are too various for another. There were, for instance, men like Elias Howe and Cyrus McCormick who developed new kinds of machines. There were men like Samuel Slater and Arthur Scholfield in the textile industry, who organized novel devices and processes to produce the factory system. Benjamin Latrobe and Nicholas Roosevelt put steamboats on the western rivers.

This narrative, as arbitrarily limited, has found no place even for the most illustrious, like Robert Fulton or James Stevens. And then there is the endless list of those less familiar who collectively made remarkable contributions, such men as James Renwick or Charles Haswell or Charles Ellet.

And finally, not enough has been said about those dominant elements: the railroads, which were the agent of "a social, economic and moral revolution," and the steam engine, the first great modern prime mover.

Still, in spite of such imperfections and limitations in the narrative, there are things to be found in the lives of John Jervis and John Fritz that were held, in varying degree, in common by all men who made and built things in the first half of the last century. Conditions stated or implied by their experience can be used as generally applying in a consideration of the state of the art in those days.

Take, as a simple and obvious thing to begin with, the matter of hard work. As already noted, Jervis, late in his career, went abroad for a month. While there, he looked at bridges and canals and railroads. That seems to have been the extent of his diversionary activity. As he said, engineers should be "so immersed in what they were doing that they would have no occasion to seek other sources of amusement." Fritz left Cambria twice in five years, once to look for better ore near Pittsburgh and once to persuade the owners in Philadelphia to continue the company. This was all in accordance with the custom of the times and the sanctions of the controlling Protestant ethic ("for him that doth not work must surely die"), but it does seem that engineers, in response to special circumstances, worked harder than most.

They worked hard because the task was great—to turn a wilderness if not into a paradise at least into a going concern. They worked hard because they found themselves almost invariably in precarious situations, only a step or two ahead of failure. To build a canal, a railroad, an iron mill—new things in this country—required dollars and management that knew what it was doing, and there was not enough of either to go round. So the difference had to be made up by acts of the will and in the sweat of their faces. They worked hard because nothing else in the early days—a gear wheel, a steam fitting, a propeller shaft, even so simple a thing as a furnace grate—worked very well. It was not a matter of ordinary maintenance; it was fixing broken things two twelve-hour shifts twenty-four hours a day. They worked hard because they were dealing with sizes, weights, and energies—a three-hundred-mile canal, five hundred pounds of molten metal, steam—that were outside any previous experience. In scale and play of forces the context surrounding their endeavors was always insufficiently understood. So, at all times, they were under the necessity to learn more. They worked hard too because whether in the wilderness or the odd new community of the factory, they were removed from the customary rites and routines of life and so sought fuller definition of themselves in further work.

It is interesting to reflect on the way in which all this energy was released to do work along the westward course of empire. A canal passing through Rome, New York, a furnace built near Londonderry, Pennsylvania, a railroad in the Berkshires drew boys off the surrounding farms. Thus energy locked up for a century or more in the enclosing cycle of growing and harvesting small crops was discharged directly into the expanding economy. In the form of physical and intellectual power applied to building and making things, it acted with explosive force upon the whole society.

Most of this energy went, of course, into doing, but a good deal of it, as has been suggested earlier, went into learning, which in those days was almost totally also a function of doing. Fritz, for example, acquired his education in the iron trade exclusively by action and observation. When Jervis became a resident engineer on the Erie Canal he had read the Bible, Calvin's *Institutes,* and a remarkable article on waterworks in the *Edinburgh Encyclopedia,* but what he knew about canals he had learned by three years of labor on the canal. This was probably, given the conditions, the best way to learn. Indeed, an old friend of Fritz said, in reviewing his career, "Let us rejoice that there were no universities and hardly any schools in reach of Chester County, Pennsylvania," while Fritz was growing up. He was thus free to find out about the practices of the iron trade without the disabling influence of theoretical considerations. This is a hard saying, but there is probably something in it, especially for those times. When Jervis went to build the Delaware and Hudson Canal, he found that a man who had been to both Harvard and Yale had made some preliminary surveys and constructions. The first thing Fritz had to do was to rip out all these installations.

The fact is that there were not available at that time many general ideas or theoretical considerations that would help in building and making new things. Men derived useful procedures—rules of thumb—from repeated experience and, given the materials and forces they worked with, these ordinarily served. And even if a man knew something of what was known beyond common practice it probably would not help much. For instance, Fritz spoke frequently of his frustration at not knowing what made iron cold short. Had he tried a little harder he might have found out, because a man in Germany had discovered fifty years earlier that the cause was an excess of phosphorus. But the fact is that if Fritz had learned this it would not have done him much good. There were so many other things that were not known about the chemistry of iron in those days that this single piece of information could not have been put to very good use.

What was true of iron was equally true of other related matters. Men building things proceeded in ignorance of how much a locomotive could pull, how much a beam could bear, how much water flowed through a channel at a given speed. So the way they learned was to begin at the simplest end of

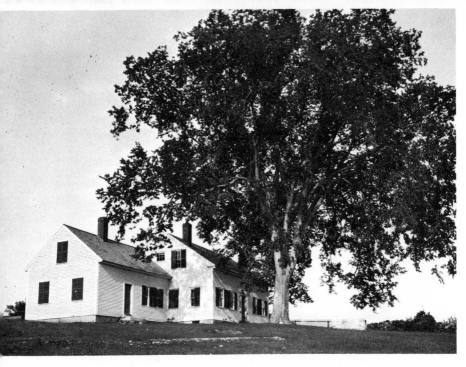

What could be done with wood, hand tools, and native
wit 200 years ago. New Hampshire farm houses. Photo-
graphs taken by Robert S. Morison in 1884.

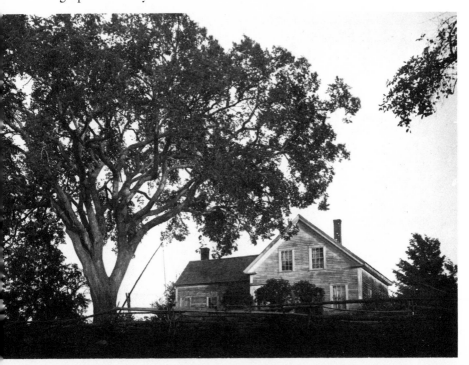

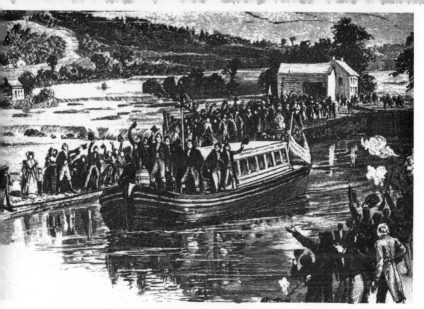

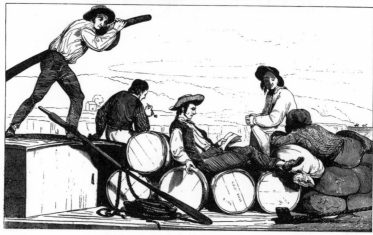

The impact
of technology
one hundred and fifty
years ago. Scenes on
the Erie Canal.

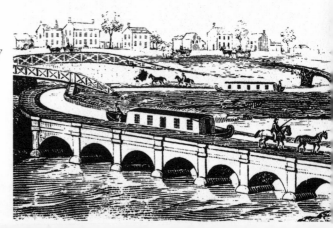

How to make a locomotive go round a curve

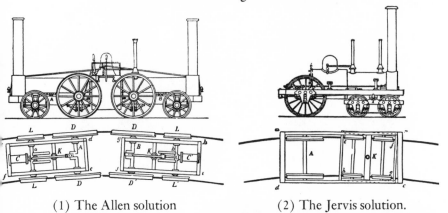

(1) The Allen solution   (2) The Jervis solution.

A parlor car in 1890

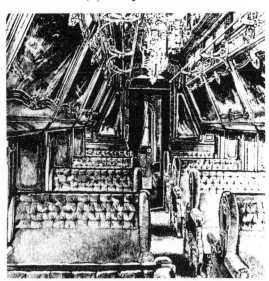

A contemporary train.

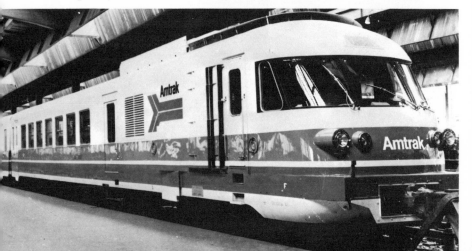

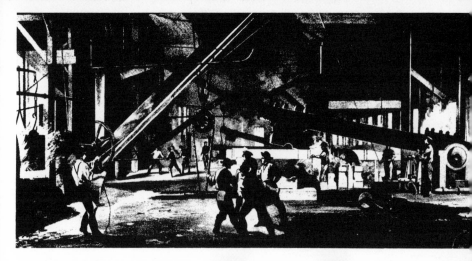

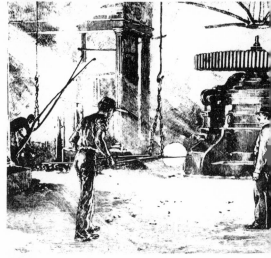

Working metal — 1880.

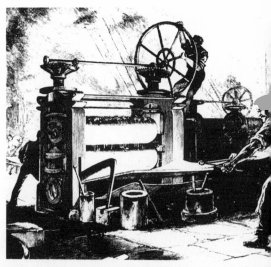

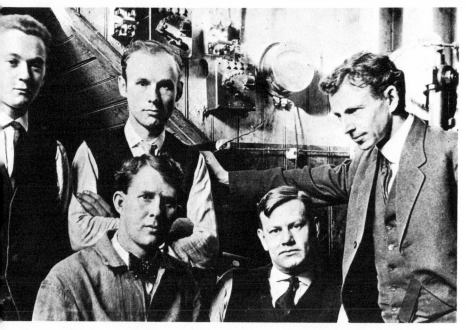

Dr. William D. Coolidge (right) and the "ductile tungsten group" at the General Electric Research Laboratory in 1911. From left: unidentified man, Leonard Dempster, Johnson Hendry, and George Hotaling.

Dr. Irving Langmuir, Sir Joseph J. Thomson, the famous English physicist, and Dr. William D. Coolidge inspect a pliotron, an early high-vacuum tube invented at the General Electric Research Laboratory.

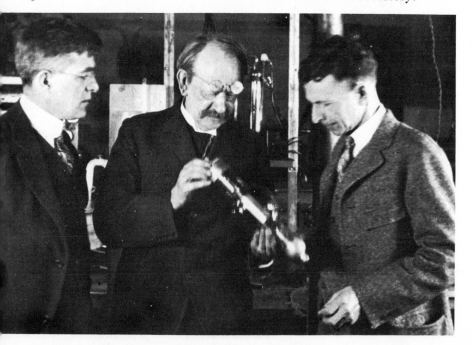

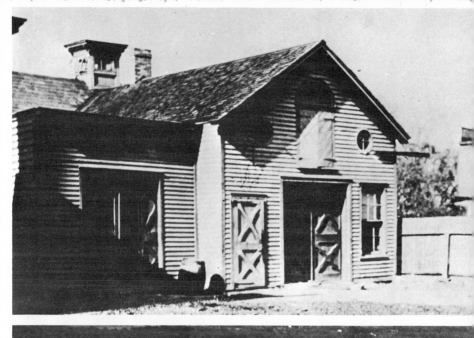

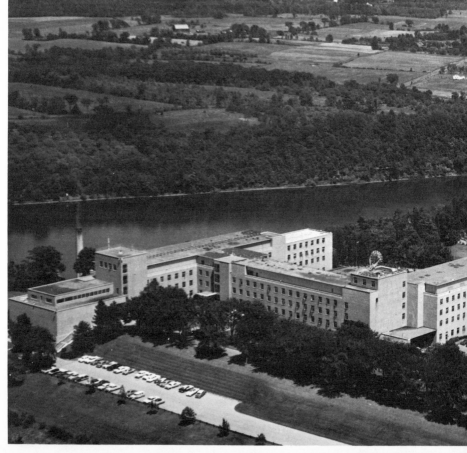

The first General Electric Laboratory, 1900.
A stable behind the house of Charles P. Steinmetz.

The present General Electric Laboratory in Schenectady.

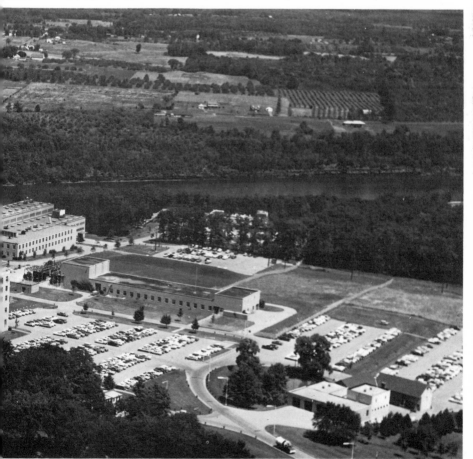

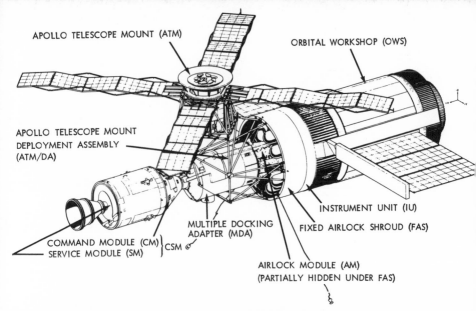

APOLLO TELESCOPE MOUNT (ATM)

ORBITAL WORKSHOP (OWS)

APOLLO TELESCOPE MOUNT
DEPLOYMENT ASSEMBLY
(ATM/DA)

INSTRUMENT UNIT (IU)

MULTIPLE DOCKING
ADAPTER (MDA)

FIXED AIRLOCK SHROUD (FAS)

COMMAND MODULE (CM)
SERVICE MODULE (SM) } CSM

AIRLOCK MODULE (AM)
(PARTIALLY HIDDEN UNDER FAS)

Space craft.

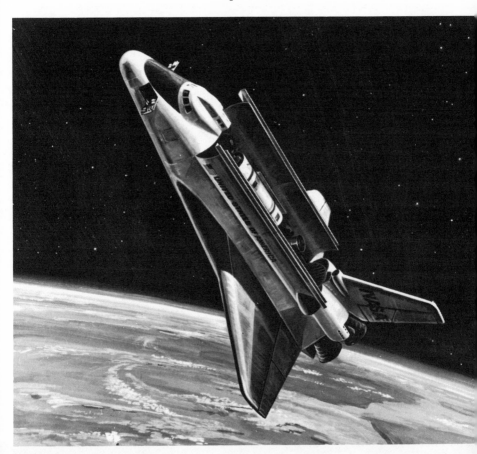

things—as an axeman for a surveying team or an apprentice at a blacksmith's forge—and proceed upward through increasing degrees of difficulty until they ended by building an aqueduct or a three high rail mill. Along the way they discarded the things that did not work and kept the things that did. And at each stage—partly from ignorance and partly from a desire to learn more—they had to try things that might not work in the hope of discovering things that would work better. In other words, they took risks.

They took the same kind of risks that artists take. Both engineers and artists extract certain resources from a natural surrounding and organize these resources into a scheme designed to fulfill a particular intent. This intent is planned to increase the utility or meaning that the resources possessed in the natural state. It does not matter that the materials are different—how, on the one hand, light falls along a seaside; what, on the other, is the expansive power of steam—the problem of organization remains the same. Things have to be put together in a way that makes sense, that will work. In a time when engineers knew as little, in a provable way, about the expansiveness of steam as an artist will ever know, in a provable way, about how light looks when it falls, the power to organize a new and interesting scheme lay not so much in the mind working within rules of thumb or unsubstantial theory as in the imagination—the intuition—that was prepared to seek operating connections between unfamiliar things.

One other aspect of the course of learning is worth notice here. The rate of advance through the increasing degrees of difficulty was, usually, matched by higher levels of competence. At the end a man knew a good deal. He understood not only the parts but how the parts fitted into the whole. Fritz, for example, emerged from his schooling in the iron trade acquainted with everything that happened from the time the metal came mixed with the ore until it emerged in the finished rail. That command of the total process was what it meant to be called an ironmaster.

From such a course of instruction the early engineers became something more than masters of their trade. They came away from their varied experiences, more often than not, as distinct personalities. Of course, like race horses and generals, they came in different shapes and sizes. John Childe, who was one of the best of them, was as open, eager, and naturally good as an Eagle Scout is supposed to be. Benjamin Wright, the father of them all, was as suave and sophisticated in the affiars of men as any archbishop. Charles Ellet, "the Brunel of America," who built the longest bridge span in the world in 1849, was a spare, withdrawn spirit in his condemnation of other men's foibles or incompetence. But when taken together, one can find among these engineers enough common elements to suggest, at least, a type.

It was, of course, an age in which it was usually possible by the conventions of the embalmer's art to arrange the illustrious dead in the posture of nature's noblemen. Hard-working, God-fearing, high-minded, open-hearted. So it is not surprising that the reports on the early engineers that come down to us fall, ordinarily, within these generous parameters. It is more to the point that such reports seem to contain a good deal of truth. Later research can only confirm that these men were, by and large, very decent human beings. That, in an undemonstrative way, they often thought so themselves does not diminish the achievement, nor does the fact that it is easier to sustain an elevated outlook if one works more with things than men and works, for the most part, on one's own.

Decency usually suggests, unfortunately, sobriety; and sober they were. In the letters, anecdotes, and memoirs there is not much humor, less wit, and very little hail-fellow-well-met. What does come through is respect for the possibilities of mankind, especially that part of mankind which fulfills its obligations and thinks clearly, and also a willingness to assign, in rather strict apportionment, credit to individuals when credit was due. But on the whole men seemed rather less important than certain often described abstract virtues— honesty, accuracy, fidelity. One of the type had carved on his tombstone only the word "VERITAS," and truth in structure is what they had all learned to live by. Working always with the most obvious and clearly stated conditions imposed by implacable nature, they found small use for wit, irony, or the arts of placation.

So there was a tendency for them to be set apart as Pharisees who were not like other men. And this tendency was accentuated by the attitudes of the others—promoters, owners, sidewalk superintendents, and men with theories. Some of these wanted it done on the cheap, some wanted it done exactly like the Pont Neuf or more like a work of art, some knew that it, whatever "it" was, would never work at all. A professor could raise a following by his explanation of why there would not be enough water in the Croton Aqueduct. Another man could bring a crowd to watch a bridge over the Niagara fall down when the first locomotive was put on it. (It didn't.)

Engineers in those days moved almost always through atmospheres of doubt and controversy. And it did not help very much that the thing that was said to be impossible while they were building was taken, when they had finished, to be a wonder. It is not surprising, therefore, that, having to trust their own private calculations of natural forces amid the incalculable noise of the crowd, they developed in time into independent, austere, and utterly self-confident men. The very good ones developed also not only imagination but a daring that was often concealed within prosaic rules of thumb and the prudential manner of the careful builder. But it was there. Engaged, especially in the early years, in many kinds of work that had not been done before, possessed of inadequate means and insufficient information, these engineers had to take very large chances to achieve their purpose.

What can be said of the achievement of these remarkable men? In quantitative terms—miles of canals and railroads, number of bridges, dams, and aqueducts, tons of iron, number of steam engines, mills, cookstoves, and sewing machines—the record for the first half of the last century is remarkable. The developing industrial plant astounded Europe and still seems astounding.

But there were other less impressive aspects of the case. Two seem worth some special mention. What was done was, often, not very well done. European observers frequently noticed the rudeness of our structures and the lack of what they called over and over again "the finish" of our products. For instance, our canals continued to leak, the roadbeds of our railways were badly ballasted and drained, our stoves were made of rough and often ill-fitting castings. As a case in point, the worst rail stock in England, the product used only for export, was called "American rail." And indeed our rails before the Civil War were never very good—they broke often under moderate use and wore out very quickly. As another case in point, an Englishman who was generous in his appraisal of our progress inspected the engine room of one of our celebrated river boats and vowed never to board another one of the vessels. Indeed, the statistics were all in his favor; the number of fatal explosions was a source of continuous comment, if not apparently of great concern.

A second condition that foreign observers often noticed was that beyond a point American engineering practice tended to stay the same. In the middle thirties, for instance, J. H. Stephenson came from England to get the evidence for a comprehensive report on the way we built and made things. Twenty-five years later, on the eve of the Civil War, a British colonel arrived on the same mission. Dutifully he compiled his findings and reported his conclusion that his trip had been unnecessary. What he had found was merely what his predecessor had discovered a quarter century earlier.

There is a good deal of truth in this remark. The tendency in building canals and railroads, in developing blast furnace or manufacturing practice was to try to establish procedures that worked well enough and then to stay with them. Our cars and coaches remained much the same for twenty-five years; once the three high rail mill was introduced it became a fixture; as soon as the iron rail was agreed upon it was standardized in spite of the fact that it was not a very good rail.

Much the same causes appear to have produced these two characteristics that so impressed foreign observers. One was economic; the supply of money was small and the labor costs were high, so the tendency always was to build, originally, as cheaply as possible. This meant cutting corners and using the methods most familiar to an untrained labor force. One was social; as Tocqueville pointed out, in a country where everyone was assumed to be as good as everyone else, everyone should share in the same things. This meant that quantity was more important than quality. It was more important that most people should have an ill-fitting cook stove than that a few people should have good ones. This went very deep in the national consciousness. While the British were building a limited number of elegant railway coaches, the Americans turned out a large number of big, uneconomic, not very well built cars. By the same token it seemed sensible to make a great many inferior rails so that more people could ride shorter distances. This social factor, as Tocqueville predicted it would, has profoundly affected the character of

American engineering right up the present. The most famous automobile in British history is the Rolls Royce; in this country it is the Model T.

One other cause was geography, or perhaps size and time. When the railroad was opened between Liverpool and Manchester in 1830 the structure of activity in a well-settled region, indeed in some sort in a whole nation, was dramatically changed. The construction of the Mohawk and Hudson, about the same length at about the same time, introduced small differences in a rural area which became significant changes only when this small road was in time connected with a series of other small roads. Our early engineers were engaged in opening up a continent which contained huge tracts of wilderness. To even begin to exert the influence of the Manchester-Liverpool canal, men had to construct a waterway eighteen times as long. To work on such heroic scales under the pressure of social, political, and economic urgencies meant that men did not ordinarily take the time to build for the ages, let alone to give their work the proper finish so attractive to those abroad.

The final and most interesting and perhaps governing cause for the limiting characteristics in American engineering was intellectual. What John Jervis, starting out as a target man in a surveying team, perceived as the surrounding mysteries of a great field remained for the most part during this period mysterious. He and his fellows followed their hard-learned practices without the reinforcement of supporting theory. Jervis, it may be recalled, always searched for the generality—a formula for water's flow, an equation for tractive force—that would enlarge his understanding of the specific he was working on. Such searches made him—as a mind—more interesting than most of his contemporaries and possibly—as a practitioner—the best of them. But in his pro-

fessional life he never could acquire enough of that generalized understanding which, framed in a theoretical scheme,
enables an engineer to advance much beyond what soldiers
call a previously prepared position. By the force of his intuition he could achieve novel and elegant rearrangements of
what he had discovered in practice. But what he had discovered in that way he could not mix with what the great Coulomb called the *"mélange de calcul et physique,"* without
which Coulomb thought engineering became a bore and certainly tended to remain in the same place. What separated
Jervis and his fellows from those who came after them was
that they had no real entry into the *mélange*. When in the
years following the Civil War engineers gained access to that
steadily developing mixture, the field of engineering changed
and so did the world.

It does not seem, in conclusion, that these early engineers
were ever bored. Perhaps it is more accurate to say that if the
restrictions of their stabilized procedures became dullingly
familiar they found ways around the boredom into continuing excitement. What they had learned on the job could, if
long continued in the same place, become monotony, but
when applied to other jobs of increasing degrees of difficulty,
it became continually exhilarating. They moved—all the
good ones—as Jervis and Fritz did—from one place to another and found the exciting challenge of longer spans,
steeper grades, more powerful engines, more sophisticated
machinery. The task of maintenance was distasteful to them;
the simple duplication of building procedures in familiar surroundings was a job for the journeyman; but the application
of those procedures in strange and difficult places, such as
Russia and South America, was utterly satisfying. And so
they continually sought out strange and difficult new places
in the wilderness.

And in so doing they laid the sound foundations for the industrial state that was to follow them. In so doing also they discovered not only the fulfillment of their own energies, but the satisfactory sense that they were fulfilling the most obvious and fundamental needs of the nation. As John Childe said in his exhuberant way, it was just a marvelous time to be alive and to be an engineer.

PART

II

Ideas Come to Power

CHAPTER 6

Plumbing the Reservoirs
of Knowledge

WHEN John Jervis and Horatio Allen met in Albany in July 1831 to discuss how to build a locomotive that would go around a curve without wearing out the rails, they were taking on a problem that was profoundly troubling to everyone in the infant industry. During those summer days they looked at pictures in British magazines, drew sketches, made small models, and argued over their differing propositions. By the coming of autumn Allen decided that his older friend was irrevocably committed to "a halfway measure." He therefore went back to the South with his decision to build his own eight-wheeler. Jervis remained to put the finishing touches on his design for an engine with the forward four-wheel swivel truck. Late in November he took his specifications to the West Point Foundry Association, a small shop that made and repaired all kinds of metal things. In the middle of the following year the Experiment was delivered to

the Mohawk and Hudson Railroad. This engine was the pro-
totype for "that first and most fundamental advance" in locomotive design.

What Jervis and Allen were doing in those months was a
primitive exercise in what is now called research and development. By their efforts they solved the problem that had
been blocking the growth of the entire industry. The money
spent on this exercise, including the cost of the engine, came
to about $7,000. The time used up was somewhere around
five man years.

A few years ago Brockway McMillan, undersecretary of
the United States air force, described some of the quantitative changes that have occurred within this process of research and development. In the making of a new set of instruments for the air arm, he said, "design, development,
fabrication and test of prototypes"—quite apart from any
fundamental research—"takes 10,000 to 20,000 man years of
effort." And these man years, he continued with unassailable
logic, could not, simultaneously, be spent on developing
some alternative system. In fact, things being what they
were, he did not believe that anyone in this country was giving very many man hours to the search for other ways to obtain the ends desired.

James Fisk, when he was president of the Bell Telephone
Laboratories, gave a fuller explanation of the way in which
all these man years are spent in the research and development process of today. At the Bell Laboratories there is a
population all told—professional, technical, and staff—of
about fourteen thousand men and women. About seven
hundred of these are doctors of philosophy. Most of these
fourteen thousand people spend their time in the region
where Jervis and Allen were working in the summer of 1831,
that is, they seek to develop and design mechanisms that will
perform desired functions efficiently. But they are supported

in their labors in ways that Jervis and Allen were not. At the Bell Laboratories there is a group of people that does what Fisk calls "unprogrammed and unscheduled research." They are free to investigate the conditions and reactions of nature as their interest or curiosity determines. The object of their searches is to supply "a reservoir of new knowledge and new understanding." Upon this reservoir those in development and design draw to obtain not only a more complete view of the conditions imposed by nature on the problems set for them but also a clearer perception of the best kind of structure for the mechanisms they are trying to create. In other words, these men at their specified tasks are surrounded at all times by supporting bodies of information and theory.

Furthermore, the tasks are often specified for them, not, as in the case of Jervis and Allen, by a real locomotive that actually bounced, but by the informed prescience of yet another group of men. This group, called at the Bell Laboratories "the systems engineering organization," exists, Mr. Fisk said, "to consider the content of the reservoir of new knowledge awaiting application and the opportunities for its use." Put in another way, the men in systems engineering use the information and theoretical schemes developed by those in unprogrammed research to foretell what problems might be solved or what mechanisms might be created to do something that has not been done before.

The object of this whole exercise is to increase control over all the resources of nature so that new kinds of work can be done and new kinds of services rendered in the interests of man and his general welfare. As the undersecretary of the air force pointed out, such organized research, unscheduled, perhaps, but continuous, such systematic foretelling of the possible, such conscious selection of opportunities for future use, such ordered flow from concept to fabrication—all these reduce the play of chance in finding out new things and limit the search for reasonable alternatives. But these carefully contrived processes make it possible to bring to bear an imposing mass of intellectual energy (sometimes twenty thousand man years of it) at a particular point for a particular purpose.

It is obviously a considerable distance from the development of the forward swivel truck to the creation of the transistor. Between these two points lies a great tract of interesting, insufficiently explored intellectual history. The great thing to look for in that history is the way linkages were slowly developed between ideas and action. One might well begin with the French and the founding of the *Ecole des ponts et chaussées* in 1747. In that school students were given systematic instruction in the application of mathematics to the field of civil engineering. Throughout the eighteenth century men like Bélidor, Prony, Perronet, Chézy, Coulomb, and Navier sought to develop theories to guide them in their designs for bridges, retaining walls, canals, vaulting, and all kinds of structural members. Collectively they laid the foundations for much of the theoretical work done later in other countries and they demonstrated to those who followed them that it was possible "to tackle [engineering problems] by means of exact scientific methods." But progress was slow. Mixing the simple-minded making of things into the growing *mélange de calcul et physique* turned out to be a complicated business. To begin with, it is never easy to create and sustain useful fusions between two such apparently dissimilar functions. Then too, a cluster of conflicting attitudes kept getting in the way. Hard-nosed men in factories wanted to leave well enough alone. They were making stuff that sold and had small use for distracting notions about how to make other kinds of stuff. And besides, as it was often said, they were, like almost everyone else, more comfortable in their "old habits and grooves."

Then there were those on the other side who believed it was possible to think good thoughts only in conditions of sanctuary. Serious ideas had to be preserved in some sort of vacuum storage. There was a conviction, as an English magazine reported, that "the effort to break down the barrier between theory and practice" was a "vulgar" thing to do.

Throughout the last half of the nineteenth century and well into the twentieth, such conflicting attitudes of mind slowed the process of bringing general ideas and useful actions closer together. The problem of overcoming these resistances was dealt with differently in different countries, and it may be interesting as well as instructive to take a moment to examine briefly some of these alternate efforts.

In England, curiously, the desire to penetrate the barrier between theory and practice seems to have come primarily from a small number of men who had spent their lives in the sanctuaries, that is, men who had been trained or were training themselves to do research in the natural sciences. They perceived the possibility that some of the things they had discovered in the laboratory might well make their way in time into the factory. So they searched for some means to introduce systematic connection and conscious order into this process. The idea was given specific form in 1871 when Sir Oliver Lodge proposed to the British Association the creation of a new kind of national institution.

This institution was to have two divisions. The first was a testing and codifying agency designed to produce uniformity in the matter of weights and measures and to establish standards by which the properties of materials and the performances of mechanisms could be intelligently described and assessed. The second division was designed as an agency for research in the physical sciences that might lead directly to improved industrial applications. For thirty years this proposal, supported by such remarkable men of science as Clerk

Maxwell, Douglas Galton, and Lord Rayleigh, lay before the country as a topic for debate. In the discussions can be found all the confusions and conflicts of opinion that attended any search for the appropriate relation of theory to practice at that time.

Lesser figures in the university groves had no interest in such an institution. Current practice was a poor point of departure for any search for truth. Work in such an agency would bring the recognized purity of such search into damaging proximity with the "world's slow stain." As for the men in the mills and factories, they argued from their grooves that the proposed institution could in no way help them in the day's work. And anyway the "times were not propitious"; neither they nor the government would be justified in spending money "for anything beyond the needs of direct utility." And finally, if by chance such an institution did produce a finding of direct utility, it would have to be dispersed across the board, and thus no one could acquire a comparative advantage over others, which is what business is all about.

Against such propositions, the argument that an industrial society rested upon systematic testing of materials and artifacts, scrupulous maintenance of standards, and the continuous investigation of the forces of nature that might be put to public use proved insufficient for three decades. But in time the course of events gave imposing support to the advocates of the new institution.

By the 1890s it had begun to be noticed, as the editors of the English journal *Engineering* said, that "the cream had been skimmed off the body of knowledge." All that was easily available had "been appropriated," used up by recent invention. The country therefore needed all the new information it could get. "Without the knowledge and appreciation of natural laws which enable the manufacturers and constructors to

apply science, we should lose the power to originate and become in time a nation of copyists."

During the last decade of the century this lesson began to sink in, reinforced by a further perception. It was not only that old fields of information were being exhausted but that a new field was emerging—electricity, "that vast undiscovered country, stretching in luminous perspective far into the new century." Something must be done soon to equip expeditions for searches through this unfamiliar terrain. Not only would the exploration prove exhilarating in itself but "fortunate explorers would come in time to green and fruitful oases [filled] with the sweet waters of pecuniary success."

So by 1900 a good many had begun to understand what Maxwell, Galton, and Rayleigh had known long before, that systematic research into the materials and forces used by industry, whether or not it was vulgar, was certainly a good thing. It could be exciting in itself. It would turn stagnating pools of information into refreshing reservoirs of knowledge. It would put the power to originate behind the prevailing concept of Progress as mere copyists never could. And besides there was money in it. In that year, as a kind of symbolic statement of this growing recognition, the National Physical Laboratory was established. As with all symbols its value must be assessed by its power to mobilize energy in support of an agreed-upon objective. In a country of old habits and many grooves it did not serve to attract all the energy necessary to achieve immediately its novel purpose, but it was a significant point in the learning curve of the society.

In Germany, of course, the thing had been far better done. Sensing early the dangers of exhausted reservoirs and skimming cream, the Germans moved rapidly to establish the necessary jointure of theory and practice. It was achieved, in the first instance, by the joint efforts of the leading scientist,

Hermann von Helmholtz, and the leading industrialist, Werner Siemens. Together they persuaded the government to establish the Reichsanstalt in 1883. Siemens gave the land and buildings for this institution at Charlottenburg near Berlin, Helmholtz became its first director, and the government contributed a large sustaining fund. The Reichsanstalt was an institution with a technical division for the testing and development of new industrial processes and with a scientific division for pure research. There was a council composed of leading scientists, heads of observatories, delegates from the army and navy, government officials, and representatives of the principal industrial concerns. For years the annual reports and a stream of official and private papers flowing from the Reichsanstalt fortified the intellectual activity going forward in universities and industrial firms.

The life of the mind flourished not only in this collectively organized and supported institution but in the manufacturing companies of Germany as well. The Siemens works, for example, developed a research division of its own. And for a further example, the Badische Anilen Fabrik had established on the Rhine a company which in the nineties had 6,500 men, of whom 75 were chemical engineers and 148 were "scientific chemists to whose originality every scope is left."

As the new century began it became apparent that the Germans had achieved the greatest success in the systematic mixing of theory and practice in the interest of industrial development. Indeed, it must be a permanent sadness that the society that most fully understood the intellectual problems of the industrial revolution should so readily have put that understanding in the service of such misshapen assumptions and dreams of glory.

If, in comparison to England, the thing was better done in Germany, it was, for an extended period in America, hardly

done at all. For one thing, given the conditions of our early history, we were, in the beginning of our industrial development, committed to dependence on others. Whether it was ideas, processes, or machines, we tended to borrow or steal what was needed immediately. We had learned from William Weston how to level and how to puddle. Our first steam engine had been brought, in dubious exception to the laws of the mother country, to us from England by Josiah Hornblower. Samuel Slater came from abroad, quite illegally, with all the plans for a textile mill and how to build it in his head. All our procedures for making iron and many of our iron workers arrived in the early days from the old country. The first locomotives, the early rails, the design of roadbeds—all the essentials of the railroad—were importations.

Then too, as already noted, once a thing or a procedure worked well enough, we tended to stabilize machines and methods at that working level rather than to seek better solutions. The immediate needs of free and equal men moving from sea to shining sea pressed so hard upon us that we avoided the perils of experiment if what we had served to get us by the present exigency.

And finally, as those from abroad were always noticing, we seemed as uneasy as the old Romans in the presence of general ideas. "Hardly anyone in the United States devotes himself to the essentially theoretical and abstract portion of human knowledge." Fewer still cared "to dive into the deepest mysteries of nature"—that is, to do what is now called research. Such judgments have pursued us down the years. In the business of making, doing, and selling we could with our borrowed ideas and processes achieve "wonders"—greater mileages, larger tonnages, faster speeds, more of anything—but in the region of fundamental principles, abstraction, purest truths we had been a barren stock. In sum, we were very good on the old know-how but not good at all (in spite of such extraordinary exceptions as Willard Gibbs and Benjamin Pierce) on the even older *de rerum natura*.

Tocqueville, of course, observed and remarked on all this in the early days. He regretted that Americans deprived themselves of one of the justifying delights of decent civilization—"the pure desire to know," the "proud, disinterested love of what is true," the ardent search for "the abstract sources of truth." But he also had other things on his mind than the displeasing crassness of a society that rejected the pleasures of meditation on abstract and fundamental matters. He perceived, as many others before and since have not, that even the purest truth comes on for trial, in time, in the market. That is, whatever abstract treasure you find when in delight you dive into the deepest mysteries of nature someone else sometime later will put to use in the world. And since such truths have real uses, what may happen to a people who have no use for such truths? It was a question many foreign observers, from Tocqueville to Lord Bryce, put to themselves during the past century.

Tocqueville's answer was that we might be headed for trouble. Like China, without the interest in scientific inquiry, we might well lose the power to change. "By dint of close adherence to mere applications" might not Americans, like others devoid of a sense for principles and theories, reach a point where "new methods could no longer be invented and men would continue without intelligence and without art to apply scientific processes no longer understood?"

There is a portent in these words written in 1835 that was at least sustained as a real possibility during succeeding years. It is self-evident that the fundamental ideas developed during the nineteenth century about heat, electricity, the strength of materials, the origin of species, the structure of matter, and the nature of a variety of chemical reactions came from beyond our borders. And in the development of the basic processes that put many of these fundamental ideas to practical use the record is scarcely better. A good many later students of the period have, like Richard Kirby, pointed out that Europeans "originated commercial steel, reinforced concrete, radio, electrical generators and motors, the internal combustion engine, steam turbines and automobiles." And so it goes, whether the data are supplied by contemporary observers or by later scholars; we did not dive deeply into nature's mysteries. It is altogether possible that this cast of mind was imposed on us by our situation. We were engaged in the effort to organize a steadily growing society and settle a tremendous continent. This unique task, not surprisingly, fully absorbed such powers of mind and imagination as we possessed. Neither the time nor the appropriate conditions for the pure desire to know were readily available. So from the divings and imaginings of others we organized systems to produce a wide assortment of small wonders in great quantity.

The question put so often by kindly and not so kind observers hung over us for a century: What would happen when we ran out of other men's ideas? Would then that which in our early days had been looked upon as wonderful become, by endless reproduction, just a lot of unastonishing things weighing down our lives and spirits? Or could we develop such respect for abstract truths that we would begin the search for those truths ourselves and thus replenish the reservoirs to draw upon in seeking new "opportunities for use"?

Many people in the last century thought, as they looked upon the flaring open hearths, heard the clanking foundries, and watched the steady organizing of the means of production, that we must inevitably taper off at some comfortable level of the higher barbarism—mere copyists satisfied with the things we could put in the saddle, without the power to originate or change.

In the event, our course turned out quite differently. It cannot be said that we underwent a great conversion in some moment of time and set off on a search for purest truth "without attachment to results." But as time went on there began to develop in certain quarters an increasing, if grudging, respect for what was called, in carefully qualified terms, "the dignity and worth of useful knowledge." It was, as Tocqueville predicted it would be, our unmeditating practicality that came to our rescue. When we discovered that by our simple-minded plundering of the reservoirs we were using up the ideas supplied by others, we found a way to enforce the conditions of search and meditation that—if sustained over many years—would replenish the reservoirs. If we still resisted the pursuit of truth as one of the high, ennobling delights offered by civilized society, we were yet ready, when it became necessary, to conduct searches for new knowledge and new ideas that would introduce the intellectual energy that is indispensable for a vital society. And so we trained divers to explore the deepest mysteries of nature with the thought that they would in time come up with proposals that were really useful.

It cannot be said that we came by our respect for the dignity and worth of useful knowledge, as the English did, because of the repeated instruction of great investigators like Clerk Maxwell, Oliver Lodge, and Lord Rayleigh. In fact, we had no men like them. Nor did we achieve it by an early and spontaneous association, as in Germany, of our leading scientists and industrialists. We were not then ready for such a self-conscious act of union. One of our first systematic efforts to find new ideas to support new processes—that is, to join theory with practice—began, as was natural for a practical people, in a factory. The men in that factory had discovered by the last decade of the last century that they could make what they were making somewhat better only if they conducted a few expeditions into that "vast undiscovered country, stretching in luminous perspective far into the new century." They found the prospect of such explorations exhilarating and they were also not unaware that in that unknown territory there were oases filled with the sweet waters of pecuniary success. In seeking to produce an electric light bulb that would work and sell, they established an intellectual method that has dominated our industrial development ever since. How they did it is the subject of the next chapter.

CHAPTER 7

Tying Practice to Theory: The Tungsten Filament

I

EVERY NOW AND THEN an exception really does prove the rule. In 1864, William Franklin Durfee designed and constructed the mill that produced the first Bessemer steel in this country. Before he built these works, at the age of thirty, Durfee studied at the Lawrence Scientific School at Harvard, practiced in architecture, acted as city surveyor in New Bedford, and served in the legislature of Rhode Island. As a member of that body he drew up, in 1861, a petition to Congress to repeal any law that deprived any loyal "subject of the Government" of the right to bear arms. That is, he made the first formal proposal, it is said, to arm black troops. None of these things had anything to do with the steel business.

What he learned about that, he learned by himself and by taking thought. He had a method that served him well throughout his life. Joined to an "encyclopedic knowledge" of engineering history was his intuitive understanding of apparatus and his remarkable power for orderly investigation. Whether in the refining of copper, the making of horseshoe nails, or the designing of machine tools, this combination of assets kept his light "so shining a little ahead of the rest."

When in 1864 he built the first Bessemer converter at Wyandotte, Michigan, and attached to it "a steelworks analytical laboratory," he was simply institutionalizing his own intellectual methods. In so doing, he built the first industrial laboratory in this country and certainly one of the first anywhere in the world. It did not last long. Those who manned and managed the converter looked upon the laboratory at first with amazement and then with fear. One dark night they burned the whole thing down to the ground.

In later years, the steelmasters looked upon this cataclysm at the very birth of their industry as a cautionary tale. They were very careful not to let too many ideas into the work they were doing. As the greatest of them all, Andrew Carnegie, used to say, "Pioneering don't pay." No doubt they were wise in their own generation. What was needed in the steel business from 1864 to the end of the century was more steel. Taking from abroad the essentials of steelmaking—the Bessemer converter and then the open hearth furnace—those in the industry soon discovered how to build on these essentials a system of production that solved the problem of quantity. In 1864, about 15,000 tons of steel were made in this country. A quarter of a century later the figure was 10,640,000 tons. It was a remarkable achievement, a demonstration of our ability to borrow, ingeniously modify, and shrewdly organize in the interests of high volume. And the organization, once established, could be conducted without the hardships of pioneering. When the market for steel was a bottomless pit, it required no great exercise of pure reason to determine that it was better to light off another open hearth than to look for new metallurgical truths in some laboratory. Thus, many of the dominant engineering attitudes described by observers in the first half of the last century were given full and effective expression in the steel industry in the second half.

The making of the incandescent electric light is quite a different case. A simple way to begin is to say that while in 1864 no one knew very much about steel except how to make it, in 1875 a good many people knew a good deal about electricity but were not at all sure of what could be done with it. For a hundred years men had been trying things out and thinking hard in an effort to obtain a fuller understanding of "the imponderable fluid." Some of the names are Galvani, Volta, Coulomb, Davy, Ampère, Ohm, Gauss, Faraday, and Maxwell. What by their labors they had accumulated by 1875 was a considerable body of knowledge and some generalizing equations and assumptions having to do with the properties and responses of electricity. It is interesting that five years after Bessemer's discovery men were making commercial steel, while almost half a century after Faraday's demonstration of an electric motor, no one had made a serious effort to design such equipment with practical goals in mind.

For this there were several reasons. For one thing, electricity reversed the classical learning process. Men had put up buildings for a long time before they began to construct a theory of arches. They had run heat engines for a long time before they began to develop the field of thermodynamics. The customary way was to start with the thing and work out to the thought. With electricity the problem was to translate the thinking into mechanisms that did work, and that proved, in unfamiliar circumstances, hard to do. Then too, electricity was not like any of the other energies men had used—wind, falling water, even steam. Compared to these it was more subtle, more intricate and followed far more sophisticated paths of logic. So it attracted men who, at first, were far less interested in finding new ways to do work than in exploring a mysterious region. And finally, almost everything that electrical energy might do—provide heat, light, power—was already being done by other means. So sensible men in the marketplace were quite prepared to stay with what they had—coal, gas, steam.

In one area, it did become apparent that electricity had a comparative advantage over other available means. It could transmit a signal faster than a man on foot, faster than a stagecoach, and indeed faster than a locomotive. So by 1837, there was one mile of telegraph line from Euston Station to Camden Town in England. By 1843, there were eighteen miles of wire from Paddington to Slough. This line was used in 1844 to carry the news of the great queen's second son and in 1845 to contrive the arrest of John Tawell. He had poisoned a woman in Slough and then caught the train for London. As he alighted in Paddington, he was taken in by a policeman who had received a signal from Slough that had arrived considerably before the train. Such things attracted public notice. By 1868, there were sixteen thousand miles of telegraph wire in Great Britain.

In America, S. F. B. Morse in 1844 sent his celebrated rhetorical question from Washington to Baltimore. And two years later the lines extended from New York to Milwaukee and from Portland, Maine, to Louisville. Thus in one small sector of its great potential, electricity became an industry. And in this sector uninformed men went to work and began to learn enough to begin, slowly, the further exploration of the other areas.

A word more about these uninformed men, the first telegraphers. As a study in England revealed some years ago, they became a casual pool of invention. Attracted into a novel calling that prescribed odd hours, uncertain work loads, and lonely stations, they rendered a service that gave structure to society from points set somewhat apart from the normal social circuitry. To their task, by virtue of its nature, they brought restless independence and curiosity. On the job they picked up in practice a good deal of information about the characteristics of the new force that had hitherto been described for the most part in theoretical terms. So by both temperament and training they became well prepared to contribute to the search for new uses for the unfamiliar energy.

One of the first and most remarkable of these men was Thomas Alva Edison. Because he was found "addled and inadaptable," he was turned away from school within weeks of his first attendance. At home he read a great deal and tried out an infinite series of chemical mixtures. Then he served, briefly, but very profitably, as a news butcher on railroad cars. In the course of his travels, he got to know the telegraphers at the station stops, and in 1863, at the age of sixteen, he became a telegraph operator himself. Such was the preparation for a career which, in the ultimate judgment of the Congress of the United States, not only "revolutionized civilization" but, in an extraordinary calculation, contributed exactly $15,999,000,000 to the human race.

For fifteen years after 1863, Edison worked mostly in the general field of telegraphy, devising, among other things, a machine to count votes, a stock ticker, and a system for carrying four messages simultaneously on the same wire. By the middle seventies, he was well on his way to his definitive reputation as the Wizard of Menlo Park. And indeed, in a field full of uncertain potentials, he often did seem to proceed to his triumphs by a kind of laborious sorcery. Ill-prepared in mathematics, disrespectful of the boundaries set by available theory, he took on all the forces of nature with a combination, as he said rather unfairly about himself, of inspiration

(2 percent) and hard work (98 percent). The inspiration was informed by years of practice and shrewd observation; the hard work was simply amazing.

If the means by which he brought off his extraordinary effects are not wholly clear, neither is the cause for his obsessive labors. No diver into nature's deepest mysteries, caring next to nothing for the advancement of knowledge and even less for this world's goods, he would become absorbed in making something work well enough to make money. This test in the marketplace was for him, apparently, the moment of truth for his experiments. Once this was passed, he became, forthwith, absorbed in making something else.

In the year 1877, he turned his attention to the incandescent light bulb. Already there was a considerable history behind this lamp. Suffice it to say here that by 1877 men knew that a wick or filament set in a vacuum and carrying an electric current would give off light. A man named Sprengel had developed a pump that would create the necessary vacuum inside a glass bulb, but no one had yet discovered the material for a filament that could sustain itself under an electric charge for more than a few minutes. In short, the first thing that was needed in 1877 was a filament that would burn in a vacuum inside a glass bulb for an extended period and without clouding the inside of the bulb.

Edison started in search of such a filament. His program was, in effect, to try one thing after another until it worked. In all, it is said, he tried over six thousand things, including a fish line, a blade of grass, and a hair from the beard of an assistant. At last he used a charred or carbonized sewing thread, which by the afternoon of October 19, 1879, had burned for forty-five hours. This was an indication that the search for something that would work well enough was ended.

Having secured a lamp that would work, Edison then devised the second indispensable element in a stable electric lighting system—a new circuit that would produce an even flow of current at 110 volts to each lamp in the system. On New Year's Eve, 1879, a great crowd came to Menlo Park to see 500 lights burning brightly in and around the Edison laboratory.

The immediate result was wild public excitement, a complex litigation with a man in England named Swan who had arrived at about the same solution at about the same time, and an intense drive toward the making of electric light for the man in the street and his home. In such heady atmospheres, all these matters were soon resolved by the formation of the Edison General Electric Company and the building in New York by Edison and his associates of the celebrated Pearl Street central power station. On September 4, 1882, this plant came into service to supply current to sixty customers with 1,300 lamps.

By such a train of events the incandescent electric light bulb was brought to the point where it really worked. To discover how it was made to work well enough to satisfy the varying demands of both manufacturers and customers in later years, one must enter a different company of men and proceed with them along quite a different path that leads to a quite different kind of future.

I I

The place to begin is with Elihu Thomson. He went through the elementary years of schooling in Philadelphia so rapidly that at eleven he was ready for high school, two years before he could be legally accepted for further education. These two years he spent at home conducting a series of chemical and electrical experiments. It is interesting in this connection to

notice that where forty years earlier John Jervis or John Fritz
had to wait upon the accident of a canal construction or the
formality of an apprenticeship to find an outlet for their mechanical gifts, Edison and Thomson, thanks to the development first of chemistry and then of electricity, could, in the
ordinary process of growing up at home, discover for themselves early on the properties of all kinds of materials and the
character of all kinds of natural processes and reactions.
They—Edison and Thomson—were two of the first students
to enter those great attic and cellar classrooms where numberless boys, heating test tubes, constructing batteries, fool-
ing around with crystal sets, came upon their choice of a
profession.

When Thomson did get to high school—the famous Central High of Philadelphia—he so impressed his teachers that,
on graduation at the age of seventeen, he was taken on the
faculty as a member of the chemistry department. Soon, he
and Edwin Houston, a professor of natural philosophy,
began to work together in the field of electricity. Lighting
and dynamos particularly attracted the young man. Studying
with Houston, experimenting in the school laboratory, reading in the Franklin Institute, he soon learned enough to construct, in 1879, a complete arc light system for a Philadelphia
bakery. As a result of this activity he acquired several important patents, and these patents became the basis for the
founding of a company in New Britain, Connecticut, to
build dynamos.

Thomson went to Connecticut to serve as the chief engineer of the company at the age of twenty-seven. Within a
year, he had designed an arc light system "superior to any
other." His work attracted the attention of a group of men in
the shoe business in Lynn, Massachusetts, who were looking
for a way to fill an empty factory. They bought the New
Britain Company and in 1883 started the Thomson-Houston

Electric Company. For eight years Thomson was the source
of intellectual energy in this enterprise, first perfecting his
arc light system, then moving on to incandescent lights, electric motors, alternating current machinery, electric railway
equipment, resistance welding, and transformers. Supported
by his ideas, the company swiftly and successfully invaded
virtually every sector of the rapidly expanding field. In 1892,
the Thomson-Houston Company absorbed the Edison General Electric Company and became the General Electric
Company. The headquarters were shifted to Schenectady
and from that base the new corporation established a com-
manding position in the new industry.

   In obtaining the impressive results of that decade, the abil-
ities of Thomson had been joined to the gifts of a remarkable
man, Charles Albert Coffin. It was he, a shoe manufacturer
in Lynn, who had brought the electric company from Connecticut to Massachusetts. It was he who had presided over
the ten years of rapid growth; and it was he who brought the
new company to birth in 1892. He was a quiet and reserved
man who spent most of his free time reading or working in
his flower garden. He was also an acute selector of the main
chance among competing opportunities, an adroit architect of
financial structures, a masterful organizer of human energy,
and an excellent judge of men. What put him so far ahead of
others was his recognition, as a primary fact, that he was in
an industry that rested on ideas. One of the great things he
did was to create a set of conditions within which Elihu
Thomson could continue to grow as an electrical engineer.
Together in those years from 1882 to 1892, they filled in a
good many of the unknown quantities in the unfamiliar equation that was being developed to express a satisfying relationship between thought and action in the industry of that
period.

   Yet one more name must be placed in evidence before returning to the history of the incandescent light bulb. Charles Steinmetz was born in Breslau, Germany, and studied in the university of that city for six years. He early proved himself a man of parts—in physics, chemistry, medicine, and, more especially, mathematics. He was also at home with the small delights of this world—cigars, beer, late hours, talk. And further, he had a concern for the way the world was running that led him to socialism and the editorship of the *People's Voice*, published by the party in Breslau. When he was twenty-three he wrote an editorial for that paper so bold that he had to leave the country, just as he was about to receive his degree as a doctor of philosophy.

Arriving penniless in New York in 1889, he went to work as a draftsman in a firm that was designing electrical machinery. One of the problems in such machinery at the time was a loss in operating efficiency caused by hysteresis, or shifts in magnetizing force. No one understood the phenomenon. For two years, Steinmetz pursued the subject in a series of extensive investigations. In 1892, he presented two papers to the Institute of Electrical Engineers in which he set forth the nature of the phenomenon and the "laws" that governed it. With the publication of this work, he was immediately recognized as a "new thinker" of extraordinary power.

In the same year he was hired by the newly created General Electric Company to work first at Lynn and then at the new headquarters in Schenectady. There he worked for the rest of his life in the sort of independent splendor that German professors had created for themselves in their universities. He did just what he wanted to do. Sometimes he worked on things as practical as the effect of lightning on long lines and sometimes he produced concepts so esoteric that he was left in "unapproachable intellectual solitude." If what he was thinking often left his fellows some distance behind him, he was frequently among them as a presence—

reacting, informing, exciting. He had a mathematical intuition of great power and was utterly at home in the realms of theory. It is pleasing to think of this renegade socialist and compulsive poker player reaching for the farthest out abstractions from the middle of the headquarters of an American corporation that in the panic year of 1893 was having some trouble in meeting the payroll. There was no one like him—that is, there was no one in the industry of this country who thought so hard and brilliantly "without attachment to results."

But it is interesting to notice, parenthetically, that at the same time, in the city of Pittsburgh in the Westinghouse Electric Company, there was a kind of counterpart to Steinmetz. Nikola Tesla, born in Croatia, educated at Prague in mathematics and physics, employed in the telegraph service of the Austrian government, came to this country in 1884 and joined the Westinghouse firm shortly after it was formed in 1886. Gifted, picturesque, well-trained in classical physics, idiosyncratic, he loved to make things work. At Pittsburgh he spent his time on induction motors, dynamos, transformers, condensers, induction coils, and electric lights.

That two such remarkable minds, trained in such austere disciplines, stirred by excitements so obviously intellectual, should find their place in the company of what Tesla called "the rough and ready men" around them suggests a good deal about what began to happen in American industry when electricity turned out to be a useful energy.

III

We can now return to the incandescent light bulb. It was left burning in 1879 with a carbonized sewing thread as the filament. In that form it had attracted immediate public attention. Ten years later 8,000,000 bulbs were produced in this country and ten years after that, in 1900, 24,000,000 bulbs found their way to the market. Clearly, the bulb enjoyed a growing public demand even though it did not work very well in these years. It could not sustain a constant level of light, it burned out after a short period, its interior walls often blackened, and it used a good deal of electric current.

There were constant attempts to improve it and some progress. The first lamps, in 1880, used about 6 watts per candle. (A candle is a unit of luminous intensity, being the light emitted by five square millimeters of platinum at the temperature of solidification.) By 1900, the lamps were down to 3.1 watts per candle. But since it had been figured that a source of white light of perfect efficiency should consume something less than a watt per candle, there was some way to go. During this same period, there were constant efforts to improve the filament, the obvious source of most of the inefficiencies and distortion in the bulb. A great many materials—fish skin, bamboo, grass—had been tried out by a good many people in several different companies. By the turn of the century, Joseph Swan's cellulose filament seemed best but not good enough. On the continent men were trying out metal. Von Bolton was working with tantalum at the Siemens Halske plant in Germany and Alexander Just and Franz Hanaman were experimenting with powdered tungsten in Austria. So, at the start of the new century, there were, in the matter of the incandescent lamp, an imperfect solution, several very interesting technical problems, some promising investigations, a growing demand and—self-evidently—imposing rewards for the man or agency that would first come up with a bulb that burned brightly for a long time at low cost.

It was in this state of affairs that three men from the General Electric headquarters at Schenectady came one day to see Elihu Thomson at Lynn. He had remained in the Massachusetts city when the company had moved the central parts of the enterprise to New York in 1892. There he had his house and a small laboratory, where he was conducting some experiments of his own in the developing field of the x-ray. In 1894, he had become a lecturer on the faculty at the Massachusetts Institute of Technology. In spite of his separation from the main offices and his increasing engagement in his own intellectual pursuits, he remained, as a consultant, a powerful influence in the affairs of the company he had helped to found.

The three men who came to see him in 1900 proposed the creation within the company of a laboratory to do fundamental research in physical science. Thomson was thoroughly sympathetic and supportive. For one thing, he had, during the previous decade, developed a prudential concern that has a familiar ring. So much new industrial application was taking place that he could foresee the time when the reservoir of available scientific ideas would be used up. Some systematic effort at replenishment had to take place.

For another thing, he looked upon the investigation of nature as a calling, an exercise exciting both the intellectual and the moral capacities of man. He tried once to put this feeling in the unfamiliar medium of a poem and the intensity of the commitment burns right through the secondhand phrasing. So he told the three that they could do no better thing than to create a laboratory separate "from all operations and commerical pressures where men could ask whatever questions of nature they could devise."

That, in one synoptic version, is the way the laboratory at the General Electric Company got started. It must be taken, even as a concept, as an extraordinary achievement. At the worst, the industrial surrounding was still a scene, as Karl Marx had said a little earlier, of "intellectual desolation." At the best, a contemporary remarked, it was a time when "the interesting lives of a few American inventors had made us feel we could go on indefinitely with a few engineering short-cuts."

The search for causality in the history of policies and ideas is a slippery business, and why that laboratory was created at that time and place may never be altogether clear. Indeed, there are several accounts, all at some variance with the one given above, of matters such as who thought of it first, who said what to whom and in what sequence. On the questions of personal priority and the exact evolutionary process of the definition of the idea, the evidence is, on the whole, derived from hearsay or later recollection. In any general sense, such questions are without much significance. More interesting is that all these men, by coming together in the service of a commercial enterprise, created an atmosphere in which it was possible to think of a place where men could ask what-ever questions of nature they could devise.

That the laboratory was, obviously, a coalition of different forces and interests is well demonstrated in the persons of the three men who came to visit Thomson at Lynn. One was Edwin Rice, an old student of Thomson at Central High School, later his assistant at Lynn. In 1900, he was the tech-nical director of the company and as such was primarily con-cerned with achieving reliability and uniformity in the things produced. Another was Albert G. Davis, manager of the pat-ent department. He brought the sense of urgency to the situ-ation. He hoped to find a way to make better light bulbs before Swan in England, Von Bolton in Germany, or Just and Hanaman in Austria did. And the third was Steinmetz, who had only a casual interest in incandescence. He was moved by curiosity. Just by being there, he was a symbolic demonstration, as he had been all along, that the General Electric Company did not know enough and had to find out more about what it was doing. The concept of the laboratory was thus the product of a conjunction, forced by a novel energy, of rival urges—conservative and radical, material and theoretical, practical and ideal—that was a new thing in American industry. In a way it was the finite, systematic—and inevitable—culmination of all those contradictory relationships that in the abstract had earlier bothered Coulomb, Tocqueville, and Oliver Lodge. Inevitable or not, the idea at first, not surprisingly, met with resistance from the directors of the company, who had accepted the trust of providing visible returns on money invested. There was some argument before Charles Coffin and Edwin Rice convinced their board that they knew what they were doing. It was one thing to conceive of a laboratory and another to maintain the forces within it in proper balance. The three visitors had asked Thomson if he would undertake this task as director of the laboratory. He refused the post because he wished to live at his home in Swampscott near Lynn and continue his own work, but he nevertheless became a determining influence in the development of the institution. He did this, originally, by persuading Willis Whitney to become the first director.

When Willis Whitney accepted the position, he was thirty-two years old. At the same age John Jervis had assumed his first independent responsibility as chief engineer of the Delaware and Hudson and also at thirty-two John Fritz had begun his first big job as superintendent of the Cambria Iron Works. These were all turning points in remarkable careers. How Whitney, in comparison with the other two, had prepared himself for the decisive moment tells a good deal about the changing state of the art.

Born in what was then the village of Jamestown, New York, fascinated as a boy by what he could see beneath the lenses of a neighbor's microscope, he had gone on to the

Massachusetts Institute of Technology, where he graduated in 1890. From there he went to the University of Leipzig and received the degree of doctor of philosophy in 1896. Then he returned as an instructor and assistant professor of physical chemistry on the faculty of the Massachusetts Institute of Technology. It was there that he had met his part-time colleague Elihu Thomson. When Rice first proposed to him that he take on the directorship of the laboratory at the General Electric Company, he refused. He wanted to teach. But he went to see Thomson, who held out promises of interesting intellectual opportunities. To these he added assurance of his own support as a consultant, of money, and of that classic seduction of academicians, the part-time job. Whitney succumbed and began his work in 1900.

Once a month, in the early years, Thomson went to Schenectady for a three-day visit. During those days he talked endlessly with Whitney and the others who soon joined the staff about the kind of work the laboratory might do. These were invaluable discussions—seminars—in the setting of intellectual conditions and directions. Each trip ended the same way. Thomson and Whitney would go to Keeler's Restaurant in Albany for dinner before Thomson took the night train back to Boston. They would each invariably order a Manhattan cocktail and a mushroom omelette. And then, as Whitney recalled, they would ransack the structure of heaven and earth and "deal with the materials of the universe." Through it all there burned the conviction of the older man "that the best contribution that could be made to God's will was to study and understand nature and use it correctly." And then the older man would take the train back to Boston and lie awake all night in a lower berth thinking of everything that had been discussed.

Whitney, as he often said, profited greatly by these consultations, but as a manager he had to proceed in his own way.

Starting out in a barn behind the house Steinmetz lived in, surrounded at first only by interesting problems, he soon gathered a company of men able to deal with those problems. He also created conditions in which his associates could do their best work. There seems little doubt that in the next two decades much that was done at Schenectady in electrical engineering and some parts of physics was both better done and more interesting than what was being done in those fields in any American university.

Clearly, Whitney was a shrewd judge of intellectual problems, an astute selector of trained intelligence, a masterful organizer of human energy. He was, in other words, a first-class manager of an enterprise. But the great distinction of his industrial laboratory derived, in the end, from what he felt about the acts of learning and knowing.

In the year 1917, he went back to the Massachusetts Institute of Technology, to which he was devoted, to tell the members of the community how badly they were doing. The Institute was a great school for trade and industry, but no one there spent much time trying to read "the countless uncut pages of science." Even if the only point of research ("working into new levels of nature's infinite mines") was to make new engineering breakthroughs, or to make students brighter or teachers more interesting, it would be worth doing. But there were far better reasons. "Some are instinctive and as difficult of analysis as are our reasons for developing at all."

Very few in this country—in universities or out of it—seemed to understand these reasons. To explain them, he turned back to his student days at Leipzig. There he was in a community—indeed a whole society—that set store by the act of knowing simply for itself. Physicians, engineers, economists, chemists, men of the cloth searched ceaselessly and, by example, passed the spirit on to others. So when "a man has showed originality" and the power to add to what is known he becomes "wie ein Gott." "Do not," he said, "make a mistake here of laughing at the funny foreign facts. Maybe *we* are funny. . . . When I made my doctor in Germany, a laurel wreath was put at my place at table. In America, I should have had to buy a box of cigars for the boys."

Such was the spirit Willis Whitney brought to Schenectady in the year 1900. There was also at work, within the company at that time, the influence of other principalities, powers, and things present. They all had legitimate, even superior, claims. The problem for Whitney was not how to resist or bypass or proceed in spite of these rival interests, but how to put his spirit among them as a leaven. How he succeeded in solving this problem can best be demonstrated by one more return to the subject of the incandescent lamp.

I V

On one of his early trips to Schenectady Thomson had suggested to Whitney that he take a look at filaments. This was a very good idea. As one of my colleagues has said, "It is one of the great subjects, there ought to be a book about it." And indeed Kurt Vonnegut has made it the central concern in one of his funniest and most interesting short stories. The book would probably begin with Volta and Davey and come down through a series of the major developments in the evolving understanding of the whole field of electricity. At the time Thomson spoke, it will be remembered, the principal source of the filament in incandescent lamps was carbonized cellulose, and it did not work very well. So to the intellectual interest of the subject was added commercial concern.

One of the first things Whitney had done when he arrived in Schenectady was to build a small, high-temperature furnace. It was his original instrument for experimentation. Into it he had put a good many different kinds of materials and substances just to see what would happen to them under the influence of extreme heat. One of the things he had put into the furnace was a carbonized cellulose filament. On removing it, he discovered that the filament had changed its character, had become, in effect, metalized. In that form, he further discovered, it could convert electrical charges into light more efficiently and sustain the light for a longer time. What he had done increased the economy of the lamp's performance, it was estimated, by 17 percent, or to 2.5 watts per candle. This gave the General Electric Company a significant competitive advantage in the market. So, at a cost of a million dollars, they built a new plant to manufacture these GEM lamps. So far, so good.

But not quite good enough. If a metalized filament was better than a carbonized cellulose filament, a filament that was really metal would, no doubt, be best of all. At least it was a possibility worth thinking about, and in 1905, even before the GEM lamp was in production, Whitney asked William D. Coolidge to come to Schenectady to think about it.

Coolidge, like Whitney, was of the new dispensation. He had been born on a farm in Hudson, Massachusetts, and had gone through the public schools there. He had then worked his way through the Massachusetts Institute of Technology and from there had gone for three years to the University of Leipzig, where he obtained a Ph.D. degree. He then returned to the faculty of the Massachusetts Institute of Technology. He was a physical chemist, and when he went to the General Electric Company, he was thirty-two years old. Like Whitney before him, he went with some doubts and reservations into this new world, and like Whitney also, he had been persuaded by a part-time agreement, by the promise of interesting opportunities for experiment, and by a salary twice that which he was receiving as a faculty member.

When he arrived at Schenectady, Coolidge determined to investigate the possibility of using tungsten as the source for filaments. Since it has the highest melting point of any metal— 3,382°—its advantages for the intended purpose are self-evident. But it has some complicating disadvantages. It is very hard and appears, upon reduction of the oxide by hydrogen, in its purest form as a powder. At the time Coolidge began work, Just and Hanaman in Austria had mixed this powder with sugar and gum arabic and had passed the mixture through repeated heating and drawing processes. What they had obtained was pure tungsten in a sintered form. That means they had a coherent mass of metal in which the constituent particles clung tightly to each other but were not fused together. Out of this material, the Austrians had made a filament that was very efficient, but that did not last long. Its brief life expectancy was commercially unacceptable.

The problem was to replace this sintered tungsten with a tungsten that was ductile—that is, that could be "drawn out permanently," as into a thread. In such form it seemed reasonable to expect one could take advantage of the metal's resistance to heat while extending significantly its life expectancy.

As he started the search for ductility, the whole thing seemed to Coolidge "very unpromising," indeed "pretty nearly hopeless." For one thing, tungsten was very hard to work. It was so hard it broke files and at ordinary temperatures it was very brittle. Beyond that, in the periodic table "it belonged to a family of metals no member of which had ever been brought into this ductile state." What supported him in the early stages were three things. He knew a good deal about other metals and he knew, as any old time blacksmith did, that most metals increase in ductility as they ap-

proach the pure state and as they are subjected to intensive
"working" or pounding. Then, from his professional training, he knew a good deal about how to put order and system
into an investigation. And, finally, every day Willis Whitney
came into the laboratory to look into the state of the search
and to ask Coolidge if he was having fun. "Fun" was a favor-
ite word of the director and those in the laboratory came in
time to realize that the question meant, "Are you still working on that problem no one else has found the answer to?"
which in turn meant, "Are you still engaged in the most exciting exercise there is in life?"

In pursuit of such fun, Coolidge began by trying to find
out more about tungsten than anyone had learned in the 150
years since it had been identified. He did this by subjecting
the metal to stages of gradually increasing heat. At each stage
he took samples of the product and worked them by "swaging, rolling and drawing." Drawing means pushing the metal
through small holes, diamond-edged dies. Rolling means
what it sounds like—passing the metal between the small rollers of a jeweler's apparatus. Swaging is simply beating the
metal according to plan. Coolidge developed and built a machine to do this that delivered 10,000 well-aimed blows in a
minute. Each sample, after subjection to such carefully arranged processes of heating and working, was carefully analyzed to note changes in chemistry and structure. The reports and records of observation grew amazingly, and so did
the understanding of tungsten.

Then Coolidge began mixing the metal with other substances to see what happened. Again it was a long, carefully
plotted series with more records and reports. Some way
along in the series, he suspended tungsten powder in an
amalgam of bismuth, cadmium, and mercury. He then
passed the resulting substance through tiny dies—drawing
it—and obtained a silvery pliable wire. At that time, he

thought he had reached ductility and the search was over. But when a current was passed through this wire the mercury, cadmium, and bismuth distilled out, leaving, unfortunately, a nonductile tungsten. But it also proved to be tungsten in the purest state he had yet produced.

To his delight, this tungsten could be worked at temperatures well below redness. He therefore made new machines "to increase the mechanical working" and refined a process that went like this: Taking this pure tungsten at temperatures somewhat below redness he compacted it in hydraulic presses, ran it through small rollers, and hit it with multiple tiny swaging hammers. What came out were rods of tungsten about 1 millimeter in diameter. These were heated to redness and drawn through dies of descending size until the rods became wires 0.01 millimeter in diameter. These wires were then put in a vacuum and an electric current was passed through them. At the end of this process what Coolidge held in his hand was ductile tungsten thread-filaments.

The lamp that came from these endeavors got the efficiency up to one watt per candle and extended the life of the bulb—it was claimed—twenty-seven times. Within five years—by 1914—85 percent of all lamps were made from tungsten. To achieve this end Coolidge had worked four years, supported by a staff that grew to twenty research chemists and a substantial number of technical assistants. The effort of this exercise, it was said, put lines in his face for the rest of his life. The cost in materials, space, and machinery was about $150,000 and the scrapping of the plant and equipment the company had built to manufacture the GEM lamp.

Now, if one removes from this account of ductile tungsten all the atmospheric connotations—the degrees from M.I.T. and Leipzig, the concept of a laboratory, the band of brothers set apart from operations and commerical pressures, the very high temperatures, the exact measurements and careful observations, the precise and intricate machine designs, the tiny, exquisite end products and all that—one can see that William Coolidge was proceeding in a way not so different from the way old John Fritz tried to make good rails sixty years before—right down to the mixing of different metal substances to get a good "neutral pile" and the drawing of heated metal through apertures of descending size and observing what happened. And not so different from the way old John Jervis proceeded from wood, to brick, to dry stonework, to hydraulic cement in search of a way to build locks on the Erie Canal that would last.

Coolidge understood this himself. Many years later he wrote an account of this work which ended with the sentence: "I must say, however, that we were guided in the main by experiment itself rather than by metallurgical knowledge."

Jervis, Fritz, Coolidge shared in a similar process, trying out a lot of things until they found something that worked. That is the way of much investigation that leads to an understanding of the nature of things, but it is some distance from that search for fundamental ideas that Elihu Thomson had in mind. Still, there were differences of degree in the order and control of the work done, by Jervis and Fritz on the one hand and by Coolidge on the other, which add up, almost, to a difference in kind.

The first two had as a primary obligation the building or making of things. They exercised their independent ingenuity amid the distractions of the day's work. Their spasmodic insights, ill-supported by any kind of information, were the result, as often as not, of some accident. Coolidge worked in a system where the product was understood to be experiment. This system was designed to define and isolate problems; it generated, organized, and retained information; it mobilized trained intelligence to concentrate upon the solution to those problems. Tocqueville, it will be recalled, suggested that repeated experiments and attempts at new applications would almost certainly "bring new laws to light." The creation of the powerful system built up around Coolidge seems but a step away from Tocqueville's point.

The step to be taken leads on to Irving Langmuir. He came to the General Electric Company in 1909 just as Coolidge was finishing his work on the tungsten filament. Born in Brooklyn, he went as an undergraduate to Columbia and obtained a Ph.D. degree from the University of Göttingen. Upon his return to this country, he went to Stevens Institute to teach chemistry. When he came to Schenectady he was twenty-eight years old. On his arrival, Willis Whitney told him to look around the laboratory, find out what interested him most in the varied work that was going on, and then go to work on it himself in any way he wished to. Langmuir came back to Whitney in a few days and said that the new lamp interested him most. As a matter of fact there was still some trouble with the lamp. The tungsten filament had fulfilled all the hopes and expectations, but the interior walls of the bulb tended to blacken after limited use. A good deal of investigation in the laboratory indicated that the blackening decreased as the vacuum inside the bulb increased. So, much attention was being given to ways to reach a more complete vacuum.

None of this was of much interest to Langmuir. What delighted him, he said, were two things: first, to have a material like tungsten, which could accept very high temperatures, to work with; second, to have within the bulb a field for controlled investigation. If residual gases—imperfect vacua—produced a bad effect—blackening—here was a fine opportunity to study the effects produced by different gases introduced one by one into the bulb. What he wanted to do, he told Whitney, was simply to plot the interactions of various gases exposed at low pressures to very high temperatures in the filament. Nobody knew very much about this set of phenomena and he wanted to look into it simply "to satisfy [his] own curiosity." Whitney told him to go ahead.

He went ahead for three years. During this time he came up with some very interesting findings. First, he was able to give a fuller description than had existed theretofore of the nature of the puzzling Edison effect—the flow of current from the filament in a light bulb to a positively charged electrode set in the bulb. Second, he gave expression to what he said were the "laws that I discovered" governing heat loss through convection and conduction. Third, he provided a model for the atomic form of elementary hydrogen.

It is not necessary here to follow in any detail the elaborate path of the investigations that led to such impressive results. But several more things should be noticed that came from his work with lamps.

1. He found out that during use the tungsten filament tended to evaporate. That is, when hot the filament gave off a vapor—as water gives off steam—and this vapor deposited particles of tungsten on the walls of the bulb. Thus temperatures, not imperfect vacua, were the cause of blackening.

2. He found that the rate of evaporation varied as different gases were introduced in the bulb and that nitrogen reduced evaporation by "100 fold."

3. He found that a tungsten filament surrounded by nitrogen did not, therefore, blacken the bulb. But it suffered such a heat loss—through convection—that it used up far more electric current than a filament burning in a vacuum.

4. He then found that if he increased the diameter of the filament, he could reduce the amount of heat loss.

5. He then found that if he coiled the filament, he got the same effect as he did when he enlarged its diameter.

6. He finally found that if he used an inert gas, first nitrogen and then argon, in place of a vacuum and if he used a coiled tungsten filament, he could make a lamp that was called "a one hundred percent advance," a lamp that required one half of one watt per candle and lasted three times longer—300 hours longer—than any other.

When he understood this much, he turned his findings over to twenty-five other men, who took a year and a half to move the new lamp through the development stage and into final production. He himself continued those studies of gases, electrical discharges, reactions at low pressures and high temperatures, and atomic structures—all of which had their beginnings in his investigation of the inside of the tungsten filament lamp and led in time to his being awarded the Nobel Prize.

Of the development of the gas-filled bulb he later remarked that it was the product not of engineering but of "lots of different lines of pure scientific work." Where before men had proceeded doggedly and step by step to improve performance by improving the existing given conditions—from horsehair to tungsten, from imperfect to less imperfect vacua—he had gone by a different path until he arrived at new ideas that could then be translated into a bulb of a different design based on a different concept. No lamp existing in 1911, he said, would have gained in efficiency or life expectancy by the addition of nitrogen or argon. What had been done, he concluded, was to derive a "new kind of lamp from some new scientific principles."

V

In the history of the incandescent lamp at the General Electric Company from 1900 to 1913 there is to be discovered a simple model for the way reciprocal connections between making things and having ideas can do useful work. The model suggests the powerful effects that can be developed when applications are properly set within *le mélange de calcul et physique*. It also suggests that one can begin at either end of the process and move toward the other end—from the tungsten filament out to some "new scientific principles" or from those principles back down to the argon bulb. It suggests also the far more powerful results obtained when the connections in this reciprocal process are brought within the enforced intimacy and continuity of an organized system, that is, when the whole process is institutionalized.

Consider again the results. For twenty-one years the incandescent lamp had been stabilized at a point of interesting, promising inefficiency. Then, in half that time, the life of the lamp had been extended by 400 percent and the efficiency of its performance (reckoned in candle power per watt) improved by 700 percent. As supplementary fallout there were, on one side, some general ideas everyone could continue to use in the search for further understanding of certain physical phenomena and, on the other side, a comparative advantage that amounted almost to a monopoly for the General Electric Company.

The point of this demonstration was not lost on interested parties on the American industrial scene. Companies that worked with chemicals soon adopted the model. By 1920, Dupont, Standard Oil, Kodak, and U.S. Rubber had all established laboratories. In 1925, the American Telephone and Telegraph Company consolidated its various small, excellently manned and organized, research groups into the Bell Telephone Laboratories. The power of the model spread. By 1930 there were 1200 industrial laboratories in this country and by 1950 the figure was 2200. A good number of these, seeking merely small and temporary advantage in the market, often simply test and tinker with existing products. A somewhat smaller number confine their deeper researches to narrow channels determined by the nature of the things their parent companies make. A very significant few devote a considerable fraction of their resources (sometimes 15 to 20 percent) to the investigation of first causes. With these funds they have sought to create conditions "where men could ask whatever questions of nature they could devise." Quite often the answers discovered by these men have made fundamental contributions to our understanding of how nature works, and quite often, too, they have laid the foundation for a new product line. Which is only to suggest the efficiency of the system that has been developed to convert general ideas into goods and services.

The model for this system as derived from the work of Whitney, Coolidge, and Langmuir is not quite complete unless one adds to it those "25 other men" to whom Langmuir turned over his concept of the argon bulb. They spent a year and a half, it will be recalled, transmuting his idea into a light bulb that could be manufactured in quantity. They were working in the gap that lies between a new understanding and a new use. In the old days that gap was closed, often enough, by the intercession of some accident that excited an intelligence—Watt and the condenser, Bessemer and the converter, for instance. Sometimes it took years to achieve this random conjunction of fortune and a prepared mind.

The process as now developed seeks to close that gap in a controlled and systematic way. Using the idea to predict the possibility of the thing—Langmuir's concept as a portent of the argon lamp—the skills and energies of a trained band are mobilized to develop a thing that will work. By virtue of their understanding and training, the members of this band are prepared to drive chance out of the predetermined path that leads to the conversion of the idea into the product. By a

multiplication of their numbers—reckoned in man years—
the time span of that conversion is collapsed.

All this is called development and can be thought of as the
place where the carefree search through nature's mysteries
leaves off and purposeful dog work begins. But even the dog
work falls within an intellectual scheme. The logic of the
originating idea and of the family of ideas to which it belongs
runs right through the whole process and controls its development. Even the pitch and position of each new blade or
vane in a new kind of turbine, for instance, is designed in accordance with the dictates of recognized principles. The
work of modern development is something of a miracle of intellectual sophistication, joinery, and management.

It is in this kind of work, hidden among the statistics on
man hours, that a good many engineers are to be discovered
today. What they do is not much like what John Jervis and
John Fritz did before them. For one thing they work, more
often than not, as members of teams. For another, they tend
to work on parts of things. And for a third, they know more
about what they are doing, which tends to keep them working on the parts they know about. The structure of knowledge and administration they work within supports but also
confines. With Jervis and Fritz, it was different. The scope
of their tasks and the limitation of their resources, intellectual
and material, forced along such art, intuition, and spirit of
independence as was in them.

Of course not everyone gets lost in systematic dog work.
Edwin Land has conceived and put together his series of
progressively more amazing cameras. Stark Draper has
brought into being the intricate systems of inertial navigation. But the norm for modern engineering is more properly
to be found in that primitive model which begins with Willis
Whitney and ends with the work of the twenty-five other

men. It is, in its way, as ordered and restrictive as any assembly line must be.

On that model we have created a whole system of production that can generate very powerful effects. We can now pour into the society a continuous stream of goods and services, massive in volume, almost infinite in variety, and subtly perturbing in its changing character. Alfred North Whitehead used to say that the world had changed more in his lifetime than it had in all the years from the time of Christ to his own birth. That, when he said it, was generally understood to be the course of Progress—more things for more people to reduce the hardships of a forbidding nature. Today, as the capacity of the system still increases, that is not so clear. Those things Emerson put into the saddle have multiplied and are now riding off in all directions. Looking at it only a few weeks ago, a colleague of mine who is deep into the system said, "Everything we did or made up to 30 years ago seemed on the whole to be for good. Now, often as not, it seems to increase confusion, perhaps even to harm."

Maybe it is time to take a closer and more detached look at the system. One place to begin is with an observation made by Irving Langmuir forty years ago. The forced marches of science and the close couple developed between science and engineering have "enabled us," he said, "to solve a problem where a few years previously it was not even suspected that there was a problem." "Who knew," he asked, "that we needed the telephone or the victrola?" Henry Ford carried the idea somewhat further. The object of the system, he said, was to fill "needs the public [is] not yet conscious of." In the press to solve these problems and serve these unknown needs we have introduced so many new goods and services that we have not yet had the time to figure out what to do with them. The flood of loose things is, in places, bursting through the joinery of the Western culture so painfully put together in centuries past.

A second thing about the system is that it has its own dynamic. Where so much is now known, it is possible to give rather precise definition to things that are not known—the hollow spots in the body of knowledge. The urge is to fill these empty places, that is, in Langmuir's words, to problem solve. It goes like this: select something that is not yet known or cannot yet be done—a problem; solve it using what is already known from past experience and theory; in the solving obtain some new information that supports a prediction of some new thing that might be done under the sun; subject the prediction to an engineering feasibility study; then realize the prediction by making the new thing. What we have here is a marvelous machinery for the mass production of self-fulfilling prophecies and it appears to run by perpetual motion.

A simple model for how it works is to be found in the early development of the long lines system of the telephone. In the year 1900, it was possible to send a sustained signal on telephone wire for about one thousand miles. One of the men primarily responsible for this achievement was John Joseph Carty, the head of one of the Bell Systems' small laboratories. He was a remarkable mind and a vivid, exciting person. He used to tell those who worked with him that the thing to do was "to pick out a first class problem and overcome it." In 1910, he set himself the task of "the immediate accomplishment of universal telephony in the United States."

To thus extend the range of long-distance telephone calls, he started far back in the realm of ideas. "There was requisite a facility in mathematics and theoretical physics. The sacred books were Rayleigh, Maxwell and Heaviside." What was in those hallowed texts not only established the nature of the problems to be solved but suggested appropriate lines of attack. To mount the offensive, Carty assembled a considerable "group of distinguished scientists and engineers." What followed was "a painstaking analysis; exact formulation of questions to be solved; full consideration of every ascertainable obstacle, human or material, assembly of just the right forces and then when all was ready, a feverish onslaught quite in contrast with the slow and methodical preparations."

On January 25, 1915, the telephone line from New York to San Francisco was opened for public service. Ten months later, after a good deal of diplomatic negotiation because the French were thinking of other things in that year of Ypres and Artois, Carty put through a telephone call from Arlington, Virginia, to the Eiffel Tower.

By progressive refinements of this model, we have reached a point where, apparently, we can go almost anywhere and do almost anything. Think of the problems we have solved and the things we have done with $e = mc^2$. Think of the success we have had with another first-class problem: there are now machines that can go faster than the speed of sound. It is an extraordinary achievement. But recently it has appeared that there are attendant complications.

They have arisen, it seems, because the first-class problems have been selected, naturally, from the field of scientific puzzles or technical vexations—things not yet known or that cannot yet be done. They lie in the world of nature rather than of human being. And the solutions to them seem often to create difficulties for human beings at least as severe as those hardships that used to be imposed by nature—which the early engineering sought to mitigate. It is not so clear as it used to be in Langmuir's time that the problems solved by modern science and engineering coincide nicely with the fulfillment of needs felt or unfelt in men and women. The chances seem to be, indeed, that the stream of new artifacts, taken individually or in their sum, will not fit in dimension, scale, design, performance, or logic of its structure with the nature of human being.

There seems, in other words, to be a developing mismatch between our extending knowledge of what we can do with the materials and forces in the world around us and our older, but less certain, understanding of what we have to do to be ourselves. And in this mismatching—such is the power in our machinery and such is the confusion about our real needs—we are likely to come away losers—ground down, blown up, twisted out of shape, crammed into computer-designed compartments, bored to death.

To find some saving order where all the things we can make or do can be brought within the range of our understanding and put in the services of our needs, purposes, and affections would seem to be the next order of business. There is not so much as one could wish in the record of our past experience to assist us in dealing with this entirely new situation. But perhaps in one strange small corner of our history, something not so clear as an analog but at least as suggestive as a parable can be found to use as a point of departure in the search for a saving scheme. That is for another chapter.

CHAPTER 8

The Parable of the Ships at Sea

WHEN JOSEPH TURNER, the painter, died in 1851 he left behind him eight or nine drawings of English seaports. A French publisher decided to put them into a book and asked John Ruskin to write some informative comment for each picture. He did so. He also wrote a preface for the book in which he said something about what the sea had meant to England and something more about the kind of ship he liked and did not like. Among other things, he said:

For one thing this century will in after ages be considered to have done in a superb manner, and one thing, I think, only . . . it will always be said of us, with unabated reverence, They Built Ships of the Line.

Take it all in all a Ship of the Line is the most honorable thing that man, as a gregarious animal, has ever produced. By himself, unhelped, he can do better than ships of the line; he can make poems and pictures, and other such concentrations of what is best in him. But as a being living in flocks, and hammering out, with alternate strokes and mutual agreement, what is necessary for him in those flocks, to get or produce, the ship of the line is his first work. Into it he has put as much of his human patience, common sense, forethought, experimental philosophy, self-control, habits of order and obedience, thoroughly wrought handiwork, defiance of brute elements, careless courage, careful patriotism and calm expectation of the judgment of God as can be put into a space 300 feet long by 80 broad. And I am grateful to have lived in an age when I could see the thing so done.

About what other things made by man with his own hands—a locomotive, a factory, the DEW line—can such remarks be made? The cathedral, perhaps, but for all its glories, it seems an expression of too specialized an intention. The ship, of course, is also perhaps a special case. And also, of course, life in its ordinary detail usually falls somewhat short of the discernments of art. It is doubtful that all the jolly tars found all the things inside the wooden walls that Ruskin did. Still, for all the possible reservations and qualifications, the claims of Ruskin for the ship of the line haunt the mind. They are about what one would wish to claim for any important mechanism or technical system built by man—especially in a time when man is trying so hard to build a whole world out of mechanisms. So the ship might serve as a useful example for a further moment of consideration. How were so many parts of human being so fully realized in an artifact? How was the thing so done?

One may hazard some guesses, a few provisional surmises. Partly, it seems, it was a matter of materials. The ship was made out of wood, flax, hemp, and a little iron. Most of these things could be found on any nearby country hillside. They could be worked into shape by tools held in the hand. There was a familiarity, a naturalness, about them. Partly, too, it was a matter of size. The natural strength of the materials, unfortified by further addition or subtraction, determined the extreme dimensions of the structure. That space, 300 feet long by 80 broad, was a frame for action within which everything lay in sight, earshot, and easy reach. The scale was of human proportion. That small frame was also a system of moving parts. At each part there was work to do. So there was a division of labor. But the reciprocation among the parts was, at all times, self-evident. The set of a sail followed the pull of a rope which followed the turn of a wheel. So the division of labor did not produce a fragmentation of effort and interest. It merely gave a particular definition—indeed distinction—to each small cause in an obvious series of causes that produced a total effect. What any man did alone around one part could be seen to serve all the others and what all did together served the purpose held in common.

The purpose was to convert energy into work. Borne by water, blown by air, the vessel was sent from port to port. The ship was, thus, a demonstration of man's capacity to control some of the force of nature. But, as Publius Syrus said, "They who plough the sea do not carry the winds in their own hands." Amid the brute elements of air and water, the ship remained only a small expression of civilized intent. From the confines of their space, 300 feet long by 80 broad, men were put into direct touch with the largeness of the world around them. So the machine that brought a fraction of the power in nature under the control of men placed men at all times within a field of natural forces over which they had no control.

It is interesting, parenthetically, to notice that Frederick Jackson Turner conceived of the American frontier in somewhat the same way—as a technical system within which men worked collectively to convert some fraction of nature to their civilizing purpose while the civilization they created remained enmeshed in the processes of the surrounding wilderness. And it is interesting to notice also that in two essays on pioneer ideals Turner reported that men on the frontier found expression for almost precisely the same parts of their being as Ruskin believed were expressed in the ship of the line.

The ship, like the frontier, was a demonstration of the use of limits. Limited knowledge and limited means produced a limited intention. There was no thought of making something that would go faster than sound or farther than the pull of gravity. The designers intended to build a machine that would do as much work as possible within the restricting scales, proportions, tempos, strengths of materials, and structural simplicities imposed upon them by the knowledge and means available to them. And in the working of the machine, they discovered the greater part of themselves.

In recent times, it has seemed that neither knowledge nor means place much restriction on what can be done. So the limits must be set by the intention. At the center of the design problem today, therefore, is how to give such shape to our intentions that, in the machinery we build to do whatever work we want done, room will be found for the satisfying expression of the essential parts of our being. Such an idea, if one looks at the fractional existence imposed by drill presses, computer consoles, and lunar modules, would seem to suggest a new kind of instrumentation and a whole new set of intentions.

But if the ship of the line may be looked to as precedent, it can also be taken as portent. At the moment John Ruskin was writing his words, its very days were numbered. Too many men had been at work too long on a set of first-class problems. There was first the gun. On the ship of the line it could throw a solid ball weighing thirty-two pounds about a mile, but with every foot of flight there was a loss of accuracy and force. Nelson's great tactical dictum "no Captain who lays his ship alongside the enemy can go far wrong" was based on the insufficiency of the gun. At Trafalgar the first shot was fired at 600 yards, but within ten minutes, the fleets were fighting at close quarters—where they could hit something and where the hits did damage. About the time Ruskin was writing, men had figured out the principle of rifling. It was not long before new guns could throw with increasing accuracy ten times the weight of metal in the old round shot, and when the new shells landed—three to four miles away—they exploded with devastating force.

Then there was iron and steel. In the same year that Ruskin wrote, Sir Henry Bessemer gave his first demonstration that molten iron could be converted by a blast of air into steel and that steel could thus be made in large amounts. Soon it was discovered, as in the case of the *Monitor* and the *Merrimac*, that iron could withstand the blow of a thirty-two-pound ball at any range. So, over the wooden walls were hung curtains of metal. And then, with the production of steel in quantity, the very walls themselves were built of steel.

And then there was steam power. By the middle of the century, men had learned enough to put engines that were not very good into the hulls of large sailing vessels. But the engines were good enough so that from that time forward those who ploughed the seas could be said for the first time to have held the winds in their own hands.

In the train of the solutions to these first-class problems came, as it always does in technical matters, a whole series of very nice problems of the second class. Some were simply continuing refinements of the major elements—greater fire power, harder steel, more efficient engines. Others—many more—were forced into existence as necessary supplements to the major elements: gun mounts, elevating and training gear, telescope sights, range finders, hull design, turrets, armor plate, paddle wheels, propellers, boilers, gearing, shafting, and again and continuously propellers—two blades, four blades, six blades, or even eight blades.

As work on all these problems of the first and second order proceeded and provisional solutions were reached, the resulting products poured into the space 300 feet long by 80 broad in a random flow. Under the weight and pressure of this stream of things, the structure of the ship of the line slowly disintegrated and the good society that had developed within it simply went to pieces.

What happened in the United States Navy in these years—especially from 1865 to 1890—is a case in point. There was first of all a good deal of difficulty and danger with each new thing, as there always is in the development stage. For instance, those new steam engines were always breaking down at critical moments and the experimental boilers were often blowing up. When the Marlin vertical water tube boiler on the *Chenango* exploded on her maiden voyage, killing twenty-five members of the crew, it was only the worst in a recurring series of accidents. The same thing often happened with guns. Captain Stockton built a cannon with a fire power "terrific and incredible, certainly unknown before." On trial, it absolutely demolished a cross section of a seventy-four-gun ship of the line. On further trial, it blew up and killed the secretary of state, the secretary of the navy, a member of Congress, a naval captain, a leading citizen of the District of Columbia, and a Negro servant.

Such things, whether occurring as the occasional dramatic incident or as the ordinary breakdown that interfered with the day's work, reduced the enthusiasm of many naval officers for the changing state of things. And beyond that, and more important, was the fact that every one of the new products—whether as large as a steam engine or as small as a range finder—changed the way a piece of work was done.

And that meant a man had to change the way he worked. The naval officers thought of a good many different methods of dealing with this constantly changing situation.

One method was to act as though new things did not exist. Captain Robley Evans threw a range finder that one of his bright young men had invented overside on the grounds that it was of no use. Sadly, he probably was not so wide of the mark, for at the time there was on his ship no gun that could fire a shot accurately enough to require so precise an instrument. More significant, there was a board of officers in 1881, twenty years after the ironclad *Monitor*, that caused a whole class of vessels to be built of wood because wood was available in the navy yards and the workers in the yards knew how to make things out of wood. There was a good deal of this sort of thing in those days.

But more often the new things were accepted under certain conditions. For instance, after 1865 it became the custom to put steam engines into ships, but strict regulations were laid down governing their use. Only a fraction of time on any given cruise—a matter of specific hours—could be taken up in steaming. For the rest, the ship proceeded under sail; and if that prescribed fraction of steaming time were exceeded, the captain had to pay for the coal out of his own pocket. This matter of continuing sails was most important. It was taken as a question, in part, of economy—coal cost more than wind—and, more significantly, of moral fiber— men did not become stouthearted and self-reliant by working around pressure gauges and connecting rods.

Another example of the acceptance of the new under certain conditions has to do with the gun. By 1880, there were rifles on American ships that could throw a six-inch exploding shell at an enemy several miles away. Some time was spent in training men in the way to load and train these guns, but not much was done in the way of actual target practice. And a good deal more time was spent in training the crews to repel boarders with pikestaffs and small arms.

All this should suggest that the navy had some trouble in getting used to each particular new thing that came into the society in those years. There was a good deal more trouble in fitting these particular things into a useful system—that is, in putting them together to make a new kind of ship. An early example is the *San Jacinto*. There were great differences of opinion over the size of the cylinders in the engine, the length of the drive shaft, the design of the gears that transmitted power from the engine to the shafting, and the number of blades for the propeller. There was even more difference of opinion about how these several parts should be assembled and placed in the hull.

A board finally decided that the propeller should have six blades on the familiar theory that the more complicated the structure the more work it could do. The board members decided that the propeller shaft should be located twenty inches to one side of the center line because "they could not bring themselves to agree to any application of steam power that involved cutting a big hole for a shaft through the stern post." This decision required that the shaft project far enough behind the stern "to allow the screw to work abaft the rudder." The board finally decided to save shafting by moving the engines as far aft as possible. The *San Jacinto* was built in accordance with these decisions. At the ship's trial, it was discovered that the offset propeller produced an erratic forward motion and that since it weighed seven tons and trailed five feet out from the stern, it was "something of a menace to the safety of the ship." And it was also discovered that the engines had been set so far aft that there was no room for a man to make "adjustment or repair of the engines after they were in place."

The *San Jacinto* is a nice example of the difficulties of

building something out of unfamiliar parts. As time passed, the parts became more familiar, but the difficulties in putting them together into a satisfying whole continued. For instance, the naval officers built a ship that went so fast and shot so far they did not know what to do with her. So they made her into a receiving ship—safely anchored in a harbor—and then they laid her up altogether. At another time they laid the keels for a whole class of vessels—four double-turreted monitors—and for the next twenty years built and rebuilt and stored and then rebuilt again these ships while discussions continued over how they were to be used. In these confusing times, they tried out all kinds of ships and ideas. They built small vessels that were "floating batteries" to protect harbors. They built some ships out of wood with iron rams at the bows that were designed to destroy enemy vessels by running into them. They built ships with so many guns of different caliber that they got in the way of one another's fire. They built a small ship to lob a charge of dynamite into the coastal cities of the enemy. And they built some ships out of wood that were fast enough and had enough guns to seek out and destroy freight boats.

Along with all these various men-of-war, there was another type of vessel—heavily armored and heavily gunned—that a board of officers concluded in italics was *"absolutely needed for the defense of the country."* But the board also concluded that ships of this type should not yet be built because no one quite knew what kind of armor and what kind of gun should be used in the building.

This was a time, in other words, of disordering confusion in the United States Navy. Part of this confusion, as already indicated, was produced simply by the flow of new things. It was hard to know how to use each new part and harder still, technically, to know how to fit them all together into a new structure. But the disorder was not just the product of technological change. It was caused in greater part by the fact that the naval officers did not know what to do with what they had. There was in fact a great and raging debate about the use of naval vessels in those days. Was the purpose of men-of-war to run down freighters and so starve the enemy; was it to lie off the harbors of principal cities and defend the coastline from the attacks of the enemy at sea; was it to lie in a line along a foreign coast and blockade the commerce of the enemy; was it to show the flag in an impressive way in distant ports?

To such questions, there was not, in those days, an answer. So the naval officers did the obvious things. First, they went on building everything they could think of with the materials they had on hand. The result was a collection of ships designed to fulfill a wide variety of intentions that did not fit together in a working way as a fleet. The hope, altogether natural, was that if the performance of the parts could be improved, the whole would fit together better. So the officers set up boards to recommend improvements in the parts. There were boards on propellers, on boilers, on shells, on guns and engines and armor plate; there were boards on monitors and rams and commerce destroyers and cruisers and ironclads and ships of the first, second, and third rate. There were from 1865 to 1890 over one thousand boards looking at everything and, often, at the same thing. They were doing what is called today technological assessment— analysis of the individual elements in a system. Since most of these boards produced something less than incisive findings, since there were often minority reports, and since what one board said not infrequently contradicted what another board said, there was not much reduction of the prevailing confusion.

So the navy did another, altogether natural thing. It sought to contain all the new machines and new forces that had produced a novel and unrecognized potential within a familiar pattern. Whatever the design and intended purpose of the new vessels, they were sent out on the old cruises and missions of the ship of the line. They sailed independently along the courses of the old triangular trade set up to protect the traders in rum and molasses and to search out the traffickers in slaves. Or they sailed independently to the Mediterranean, where naval ships had earlier done great things against the Algerian pirates. Or they cruised to Halifax through waters formerly troubled by fishing disputes. It all made very little sense and continued an uncertainty in the naval service about machines and purposes that produced "a mere welter of minor excitements" since the machines were always changing.

The situation was intensified for the naval service by several other considerations. As one thing after another dropped into the space 300 feet long by 80 broad, the members of that community came to believe that all those parts of their being that had been realized in the ship of the line were "put in the course of ultimate destruction." "Lounging through the watches of a steamer, or acting as firemen and coal heavers, will not produce in a seaman that combination of boldness, strength and skill which characterized the American sailor of an elder day." Worse still, the possibility of opening an engagement at a range of five miles "would create an indisposition to close" with the enemy, a reluctance to come into direct contact with reality that would in time pervade all life. And beyond that was the possibility, as more and more things dropped into that small space, that the intention of John Ericsson would be ultimately fulfilled. After he built the *Monitor*, he hoped to construct a ship so perfect that it would remove men from the sea. This may well be the unstated premise in all machinery.

In the middle of such perplexities, ambiguities, and anxieties, Alfred Thayer Mahan wrote a book called *The Influence of Sea Power on History*. The object of a navy, he said, was to command the sea. To achieve that end, he said, it was not necessary (it was not even wise) to send vessels in all shapes and sizes all over the enormous waters to search and destroy whatever could be found afloat. What was needed was a concentration of forces, a balanced fleet. The principal element in that fleet was the largest, best protected, most heavily armed vessel that could be built—a battleship which derived its name from its predecessor, the ship of the line of battle. In support of the battleships were lesser elements, cruisers and destroyers with clearly defined missions of search, screening, and protection. All these elements in proper combination would move to action far at sea and there engage an enemy fleet. Success in this encounter would secure the integrity of the shipping lanes, protect the distant coastlines, and establish dominion over all the seas. There were countless supplementary details, but, in substance, it was about as simple as that.

What followed, considering the work was only a book, and a book of history at that, was quite surprising. For one thing, everybody who was somebody or was about to become somebody seemed to be reading Mahan's words. Lord John Fisher took the book to sea with him. A member of the Civil Service Commission in Washington named Theodore Roosevelt swirled through the pages at his usual breakneck speed and, as usual, remembered every word of it. The emperor of Germany had it on his bedside table. For men in embassies, wardrooms, chancelleries, newspaper offices, and legislative halls it became required reading. In America, the secretary of the navy traveled to Newport to close down the Naval War College, where the book had been written. On the way from Washington to Rhode Island he read enough in the volume to make him decide to keep the college open. It was also surprising that everyone who read the book seemed to understand what it was saying.

Most surprising of all was what began to happen, after publication, in the United States Navy. Within a year or two, the confusing arguments over the merits of blockade, coast defense, harbor protection, and commerce destruction ceased. Within two or three years, the problems of ship type, ship design, gun size and distribution, weight of armor, and size and composition of the fleet were all moving toward resolution. There was a great reduction in the number of boards to study the situation, but of course some remained.

Given the stated purpose and the grand design, all the disparate parts and pieces of machinery, all the technical details started to fall into place. And as that happened, all the training routines and operating procedures and even the personal feelings built up around working parts and within technical systems also fell into place. For the first time in half a century, men had a clear idea of what they were trying to do with their mechanical structures and how they might shape and use them in support of their purpose. It was a remarkable demonstration of the power that lies in a governing idea.

A parable, in the ordinary way, should be allowed to stand by itself. The conversion of the content into meanings that can be usefully applied in other circumstances is usually left up to the individual interpreter. Accordingly, correction for the differentials between a sixteen-inch gun and an IBM computer of the 370 series, or an armed force and a free society, or a ship and the real world is handed over to each reader. But as an excuse for further explication something more may be said about why this naval case has been fitted into the line of thought that is supposed to run through this book.

Briefly: Things went on well enough for the men in the naval service as long as they worked with familiar and limited means. Then gross and continuing expansion of the means threw them into a considerable confusion. At first it was simply a matter of trying to figure out how all the new apparatus worked, but then the uncertainty over the novel means extended to the ends. What were they to do with all these things that so enlarged their own capacities? For some time they hoped to solve this problem of the ends by making the means work better—improvement in the technology, as it is now called. But that simply added to the confusion. Then Mahan explained what the purpose of a navy that had all these new things should be. Given such a defined and recognized end in view, the men in the service then found they had a way to put all the forces and materials that had distracted them into a sensible system that served the intended purpose. It was a system they could manage in an informed way.

Spelling it all out—if you know the kind of war you want to fight you don't have much trouble designing and controlling the machinery. Spelling it out still further—it should work the same way if you can figure out what kind of life you want to lead. Frankenstein ingeniously came up with a marvelous creation and it did him in because he hadn't thought through what he wanted to do with it.

For a long time making marvelous creations seemed enough. Bacon put the case very well. What is true and what is useful come, in the end, to the same thing. Accurate knowledge of the universe derives not so much from speculation on the divine as from the mind doing things with the resources nature has made available. "Works themselves are of greater value as pledges of truth than as contributing to the comforts of life."

Within such sanctions and with the best intentions men like Baldwin, Jervis, Fritz, Coolidge, Whitney, and Langmuir did great things. By their works, one after another, they added to the sum of what there was to know and made more people more comfortable. In so doing they and those who came after them developed an instrumentation that proceeded from the simple to the very sophisticated. And by this means was started a stream of goods and services that flowed from scarcity toward plenitude and infinite variety and, as in the naval service, a growing confusion. Neither the accumulating truth about nature, on the one hand, nor the amplifying progression of infinitely various comforts, on the other, appears to serve as a sufficient organizing principle. Having by wit, imagination, hard work, and the best intentions produced a remarkable system for doing things for us, we now, by the same means, have to reach some agreement on what it is we want done.

CHAPTER 9

Some Notes on Visions

AND SO one comes back to the beginning and to Whitehead delivering his charge to reenact a saving vision. At almost the same time that he was doing so, William Butler Yeats made almost the same argument. "Things fall apart; the centre cannot hold . . . The best lack all conviction, while the worst/Are full of passionate intensity."

Given such conditions, as Yeats said, "Surely some revelation is at hand." Failing that, "Mere anarchy is loosed upon the world." "Mere anarchy" or "mere welter of minor excitements," it comes to the same thing in the end. These men made their points a half a century ago and suffered the fate of poets and philosophers. They were sometimes quoted in pulpits and at college commencements as the congregations and the graduating classes went out to do the work of the world.

Now these forecasts have been overtaken by events and many of those who did not read before now see that we are all running for dear life. There are those who worry about the contamination of the atmosphere. There are those who worry about the misallocation of our resources and the discovery of finite limits to the growth of our material development. There are those who worry about the alienation or the *angst* or the *anomie* or the outright doom of the post-industrial, technological, or automated man. There are those, the young, who have left the complications of their artificial surroundings to grow vegetables, raise sheep, build houses out of wood with their own hands, and otherwise make a living in blue jeans in a piney glade. There are those who seek to fight their way out of their numbing context by random acts of violence. And then there are you and me and Bindlestiff, clinging to the day's routines and our received positions because the center is not holding. The making of visions, like any other business, needs a market and one seems to be developing.

As a result, a good deal of attention is already being given to the shape of things to come. Looking ahead is now something of an infant industry. The initial products, though available in considerable variety, are not yet very reassuring. In one way or another, taken as sustaining revelations, they have significant defects. A few men, like Jacques Ellul, have looked over the future and concluded that it just won't work. Others, a good many others, have let their imaginations go on particular possibilities when some of the machines and procedures now in the development stage reach perfection. Their findings are as precisely stated and hair-raising as anything in the Book of Revelation: man as the drone in a hive designed by a computer; man as an assembly of spare parts—kidneys, pineal glands, brains; man cloned into existence as some new product of rational selection.

Others have approached the subject in more scholarly and philosophic moods. They are often very instructive about the complications of the present situation and sensitive to disturbing possibilities in the future if things go on much longer without sensible control. But their own prescriptions are stated, on the whole, in cautious generality. Daniel Bell, one of the most prominent students of these matters, is not willing, in his recent "venture in social forecasting," to go much beyond the suggestion that the next society will be "an analytic construct," a "specification of new dimensions in the social structure which the polity has to manage." And Viktor Ferkiss, one of the best men in the business, believes he can do no more than try "to point out at least a direction in which mankind must go if it is to be able to deal with the new challenges put to the social order by technological change."

More specific is the contribution of Jay Forrester and those who follow him. He has created a model of our present economic system and uses it to demonstrate his belief that the workings of that system move so rapidly toward the depletion of essential resources that very soon it will be impossible to meet the needs of the population. There are, in other words, such definite limits to our growth that we must plan a different kind of world for ourselves.

The reception of these propositions may suggest why many scholars prefer the sanctuary of ill-defined generality. A considerable hue and cry has been raised about these models. The tidiness of the conclusion has been achieved, it is said, only by the use of false assumptions and the exclusion of inconvenient variables. Whatever final judgment may be passed upon the integrity of the work, the contribution has already been considerable. Forrester attempts to deal rationally with very specific things. He thus has given a focus to and a way of thinking about all the lurid images and free-floating anxieties. In the long run the Forrester model may prove most useful simply as a pedagogical device, but that is no small thing.

Two other attempts to deal with the shape of things to come deserve some mention here. There is the scenario, an instrument being developed in industry to help in the work of forward planning. Insofar as scenarios deal with matters like the presumed GNP, the probable tax structure, and projected per capita income, these studies may be said to be tied to some realities. But in the admittedly more complicated matter of the probable state of the social psyche they leave a good deal to be desired. In a working paper for one of these exercises, I read that by 1990 competitiveness will have shifted from "the adversary I win/you lose type to something more sporting and impersonal." Also in that same year, consumers will be "hungry for trouble-free, tasteful, reliable and distinctive purchases." Aside from the fact that those who make such assertions do not appear to have much data in the bank, there is the difficulty that uppermost in the minds of those who write scenarios are such limiting concerns as whether—ten, fifteen, thirty years hence—there will still be a market for clothes driers or four-wheeled vehicles.

The final effort to think ahead is somewhat different from all the others in that it presupposes some action now, but it contains some interesting things for those who wish to enter the vision business to think about. It is the battle plan to reduce some particular salient that looks as though it could cause trouble in the future. We are, says a friend of mine, veterans of numerous wars—the war on poverty, the war on tuberculosis, the war on inflation. Hardly had he spoken (November 1973) when a little girl peered out of the pages of the *Atlantic* and asked, "Daddy, what did you do in the war against pollution?" The text went on to say that in this war there were no 4Fs and COs. All were soldiers and everyone could fight by doing things "like cleaning your spark plugs every 1,000 miles."

Great things have been done in the past by those who held the heroic view and by the massive offenses mounted in support of our peculiar position as the last best hope of earth.

But the concept of war as a way of dealing with many of our future problems does not seem very promising. For one thing, the apocalyptic call to arms does not say much, indeed anything, about the nature of the problem to be attacked. For another, the disparity between the majestic summons and the proposed combat procedures—clean your spark plugs and so forth—is enough to discourage any soldier before he has finished his basic training. And finally, and most important, the concept of war suggests a false conclusion. The conflict is to be fought, as our historical imperatives indicate, to unconditional surrender—which is to say that there are always fixed and final solutions that can be imposed on such difficulties as are caused in a technological society by an excess of carbon monoxide or an insufficiency of oil. Such is not the case. We work with limited means and within a system where one thing interacts with another. So the problems will not yield to *la guerre à l'outrance* but must be dealt with in a series of continuing adjustments and trade-offs in which everyone gets somewhat less than the optimal expectations or even than his just deserts. Of this, more later.

All the foregoing should indicate that the future is now a big topic. It should also indicate that the talk about it has not—so far—done much to prepare us to deal with the days ahead. Those scenarios, mathematical models, ventures into social forecasting, those big boneless political slogans like Project Independence do not suggest that surely some revelation is at hand. And they do not give much aid and comfort to anyone who is trying to find out how to re-create a vision. In the past, the thing was, often, somewhat better done.

The point of many of those older visions was to give an unusual structure to the available data, to describe a general aim close enough to what was possible to pass a feasibility study and far enough removed from it to open up exciting opportunities. The object was not to define what was happening but what, given the existing means, ought to happen. The point of departure was thus an assumption containing a moral intent. It was this that gave a good vision much of its attractive power; it gave a focus to the day's work that made that work more interesting or satisfying than, taken just by itself, it really was. Within that focus, perspectives were extended, sights could be elevated, and, most important, generalizing significance was assigned to individual action. There was a further source of attractive power. The aim of a good vision was set forth, as in any dream, with great specificity. Whether the point was stated literally—save France—or was cast in the symbolic form—find the grail—the rendering was detailed and precise. So much is obvious.

Less obvious is the fact that the good vision was just as concerned with and just as specific about the means as the ends. To save France, you were to start with the relief of Orleans; to get within sight of the grail, you fulfilled the regulations of the chivalric code right down to the way to take care of the horses. So, with all its expansive power, a good vision, in its specificity, in its careful connection between means and ends, in its explication of causes and effects, also imposed metes and bounds—a theory of organization, a set of limits—on human action and desire. That too was a source of its attractive power.

The last great scheme for attracting and organizing the energies of men conformed to many of the requirements for a good working vision. This was the concept of Progress that dominated the Western world for a century from the defeat of Napoleon at Waterloo to the pistol shot at Sarajevo in 1914. In its origins it departed somewhat from the traditional methodology. Instead of appearing on some spectacular occasion in a moment of time, as at Domremy, it was slowly assembled by the work of many heads and hands. And thus it fell somewhat short of exact definition. It was put forward at various times as "one increasing purpose which through the ages ran," or as "the movement of mankind onward and upward forever," or again, as a great spinning "down the ringing grooves of change."

General though these concepts were, they all did suggest what was a fairly new idea at the time—that things did not have to stay the same, that, by taking appropriate action, men could make things better. In time, confirmation for such a view was forthcoming from unexpected quarters. Darwin, asserting that no condition was constant, discovered that progress appeared more frequently than retrogression and Spencer postulated that progress was not an accident, but a necessity. In time, too, the definition of what Progress was, was brought within clearer limits. Samuel Butler gave the clue when he said in his jeering way that "progress is based on a universal innate desire on the part of every organism to live beyond its income"—that is, to raise the standard of living. As time passed that is what, increasingly, Progress was understood to mean, the multiplication of goods and services for everyone, the steady improvement of the physical conditions of life.

The means to this end were stated with appropriate specificity: duty, thrift, freedom to move out and up, and very hard work. Men acting within these sanctions soon discovered that the program produced excellent results. Their energies, miraculously amplified by all the new machinery, turned out all those goods and services that were the measure of progress in a swelling stream.

There were, of course, temporary injustices, local inequities, and episodic horrors, but on the whole, the movement was in a favoring direction. Those who had plodded their weary way, in 1800, through the short and simple annals of the poor came, as time passed, into possession of automobiles, telephones, television sets, air conditioners, credit cards, fringe benefits, oil heat, major medical contracts, electric light, old-age annuities, snowmobiles, and the forty-hour week. It was all done in the space of 150 years. By any standard, it is astounding.

It shows what can be done when human energy is released and mobilized by the power of an attracting vision, a general scheme. In fact, it probably was the very generality of the scheme that made it fit the times so well. When a bridge, a light bulb, a steel beam, or a telephone wire was understood to serve the progress of human affairs, men were set free to seek out many kinds of invention. While men had the opportunity, by taking thought, working hard, and pursuing every kind of main chance, to improve their own station, they had confirming evidence that they were also increasing the general welfare.

And now it appears that the thing has been overdone. Even before we have sufficiently increased the standard of living of every single person, we are in trouble. Slowly, it is being borne in on us that the power in the idea of Progress as simple accretion is about played out. Everyone eating his cake—all kinds of cake—and having it too; the great days when the impossible took only a little longer are over. Things fall apart and will continue to do so until a center is developed that will hold.

So how to proceed with the construction of a new scheme? As with any vision, there must be some initial assumptions. The first and great assumption is that at the center we should put ourselves. That is to say, we should begin with the idea that the technological universe should be designed to fit and serve the human dimensions. Whatever is good for us is the greatest possible good that can be allowed to General Motors or any of the other makers and shakers of modern times.

What is merely financially attractive or technically interesting must give way before the superior claims of the human condition.

That is easy to say and a good many people are now saying it. That is what the interminable discussion of values is all about. But the thought that the nature of man is to act as the controlling agency in all our arrangements introduces some very complicating elements. The fact is that while we have succeeded in making man the measure of all things, we have no very reliable codification of his own weights and measurements. What we have, for the most part, are assumed approximations supplied by philosophers, poets, historians, and men of God during the centuries past. And even these approximations are often not very helpful since they were derived from the evidence of times quite different from the present. One way of putting it is to say that even in the matter of mere operations—let alone the highest reaches of the spirit—we do not have much hard data on the performance characteristics of the human system in our strange conditions.

Take so obvious and simple a thing as work. It is something that all our days we have had to do. It has been explained in the past as everything from a curse for our first disobedience to "love made visible." Whatever the explanations, we have had, through history, to proceed in the sweat of our faces. In the course of that experience, we have learned some very bad things about work. Some have worked far too hard, some have begun far too soon, some have gone on far too long; some (in recent times an increasing number) have worked at jobs of paralyzing dullness, jobs meaningless in any way save for the payments (sometimes quite high payments) received.

The most obvious way to avoid the indignities, injustices, pains, and sorrows of all this hard labor is to get out of it. A considerable start has been made in this direction. The technical systems we have devised move toward the displacement in many kinds of work of human beings by machinery. It seems possible to look forward to a time, if we continue in this way, when there will not be very much to do.

Given our backbreaking history, it is perhaps altogether natural to proceed in the belief that it will be enough to lift the weights from all men's shoulders. Acting in this faith, we have already gone far enough to create a new thing called leisure. And we have done pretty well in thinking of ways to deal with that—snowmobiles, ten-day flights to faraway places that become steadily more like the places we left so that we may feel at home, the Green Bay Packers on Monday night, Las Vegas, campers. There is even talk of continuing education. This is all very well, but it may not serve indefinitely and it may, at best, only be treating symptoms. The fact remains that we as yet do not know much about the place of work in man's nature. Is it (even if it ceases to be stark necessity) a perennial curse, a manifestation of love, a biological need, a neurotic necessity, or just something which under certain conditions men and women like to do? And if it is a given in our nature, in what conditions can work be performed so that it is a source of satisfaction? How, in other words, can the jobs, the machines, and the technical systems be designed to fit not so much the claims of production as the requirements of human beings? To answer such a question, we need to know much more about men and work than we do now.

There are other things we need to know. The technological systems we construct move, self-evidently, toward increasing change. Man, in the past, has been differentiated from all other creatures by a remarkable capacity to accommodate. He has moved, in large part by taking thought, from the cave to the condominium, from the foot pace to the speed of sound, from hard labor to services supplied by a whole structure of invisible hands. A great question now is whether he can continue this amazing power of accommodation in a period when more and more things in his environment change more and more rapidly and when that process of change produces not only increased goods and services, but increased confusion. At what point will he simply break down as fuses blow in an overloaded system?

The technological systems move also steadily toward logicality. The machines are designed in accordance with the principles of logic; the circuits, the networks, the print-outs rest on the base of reason. That is because our technological environment derives from our scientific understanding, which explains how nature works. And nature, it turns out, miraculously works, in fundamental matters, in accordance with the rules of logic. To the extent that man thinking is man being, it is sensible to suppose that he can find comfortable accommodation in the universe he is building for himself. But he also feels, and these feelings, which are also a part of being, do not flow along the ordered paths of logic. Certainly, any re-created vision for a technological world must reflect in its design the unflinchingly rational, but how much room must be found in that design for the play of feeling? Put another way, how do we find the point beyond which man, with all his nonlogical components, cannot stand logicality?

And finally, technological systems proceed toward generality and abstraction—numbers, models, print-outs, credit cards, experience converted into pictures, and so forth. The power to abstract has been a principal resource for man in the struggle from the primal mud to the high-rise. But still much of his experience has remained literal and concrete—face to face, reaping where one sowed, building with one's own hands, judging by the actual fruits thereof, and so on.

The question here is how much abstraction can man stand, how much removal from first causes, how much action at a distance, how much translation of personal experience into attenuating resemblances or symbols, before he gets beside himself among the shadows?

These are all questions—about man and work, man and logic, man and abstraction—for which there are only dusty answers to be found in the old high culture that was built up in a different context. If one seeks to construct an ordering scheme for man's action in the new dispensation, one must seek firmer evidence on all these matters. It is not obvious how the search can be most effectively conducted, but one small precedent may suggest at least how one might begin.

Some years ago, there was a series of rather distasteful experiments undertaken in what was called sensory deprivation. In these experiments the subjects—people—were sealed off from all normal stimuli. They were supplied, in effect, with all the presumed comforts of the cocoon. In such conditions, the personalities tended to disintegrate or, perhaps more accurately, to degenerate into what a friend of mine called a vague oblong blur. The provisional conclusion was that men depended, to an unsuspected degree, upon connections with the supporting environment or, as one physiologist said, that they realized their potential only when serving as nodes in a communication network.

Such a finding has not met with a favorable response from those schooled in the thought of man as noble in reason, infinite in faculty, in apprehension how like a God. Indeed, I once watched a celebrated professor of English literature blow his not very well-designed stack when the idea was presented to him at a conference. But it does not seem ignoble to suggest that man, like any other system, is built to certain tolerances. If there are limits to his capacity to withstand an excess of nothingness, there are probable limits to his capacity to withstand an excess of logic, change, and abstraction. As a beginning in the recognition of these limits, it seems reasonable to propose a set of experiments designed to put men into conditions where exposure to such excesses reaches saturation point or, as they say in engineering, drives men to the point of refusal—that is, the point beyond which men cannot go without losing their senses or their meaning.

There is yet a further consideration in the effort to make man the center in all our future arrangements that is not so susceptible to experiment as are his responses to work, change, logic, and abstraction. That is his response to power. The word taken from the old high culture on this matter is not good. Whether it is transmitted by old saws, poetic insights, or the documented investigation of the social sciences, it all comes out about the same. "If you give him an inch he'll e'en take an ell," "power tends to corrupt and absolute power corrupts absolutely," "for each man kills the thing he loves"; "power; like a desolating pestilence, pollutes whate'er it touches," and "homo homine lupus," which is Sigmund Freud and which means "man is a wolf to man."

These are not very reassuring findings for anyone who seeks to make the condition of man the very center of a sustaining vision. And indeed it is this matter of man's response to power that poses the central question about our effort to organize a future that can satisfy or even continue. Throughout our extended past, if we were not quite sinners in the hands of an angry God, still we were always constrained to act within the strict conditions imposed by nature and our limited competence. Without sufficient knowledge or command over existing forces, we were fixed in an adversary process against our natural surroundings. In the adversary position, especially if one works from an insecure base of operations, one often behaves badly. We often did. We frequently attacked nature with small abuses and since we could never extract from her enough goods and services to go around, we were frequently dreadful to one another. The saving grace in this historic experience seems to have been not so much the mitigating force of our good intentions (though they were always there) as the fact that our knowledge and power were never enough to enable us in our acts of violence to do ultimate damage to our surroundings or ourselves.

But now the situation is changed. In our novel conditions, we may be said to have the whole world in our hands. And will we then on one fine day blow ourselves up or, as is more probable, do ourselves in amid a mere welter of minor excitements? The record suggests that such knowledge and power as we have acquired through the centuries has never been successfully contained by good intentions except from time to time. So the question of whether we can wisely administer the world we have built in our own interest lies open. The argument from experience holds that we almost certainly cannot. There is no doubt much in it.

But another line of argument suggests, at least, that we may. As Abraham Lincoln explained to his fellow citizens, we too are in a time when we cannot escape history. As with them in their perilous days, "No personal significance or insignificance can spare one or another of us. We—even we here—hold the power and bear the responsibility." Acceptance of both ends of this proposition—holding of power and bearing of responsibility—has steadied all sorts and conditions of men in all kinds of hard times before. There are particular cases from Prince Hal to Harry S. Truman. And there have been short-run demonstrations by whole societies—this country from 1775 to 1789, for instance. Today the dimension is on a grander scale. When there is the power to do almost anything, everything becomes a responsibility, but the principle is the same. Released from the adversary process, assured by what we know and can do, it is at least possible that we can steady ourselves enough to learn how to discharge wisely our novel obligation for the whole. It is more than a possibility, it is a simple necessity. So the second assumption for those seeking to re-create a sustaining vision is that the world men have managed to build is in fact under certain conditions manageable by them.

And the third assumption is like unto it. There is a school of thought which holds that in times like these power and responsibility must be reserved for the few who are equipped to decide and act in the interests of the many. The argument is that when "knowledge doubles every ten years," when the sophistication in systems increases by geometrical progression, and when the control of the forces of nature moves toward the absolute, the problems are too important (and too arcane) to be left to the generality of men. And, of course, there is a good deal in it.

The proposition is as old as our history ("Your people, sir, your people is a great beast"), and as new as the last election ("The average American is just like the child in the family"). Those who are intelligent and well-placed have a tendency to think that way whether there is only one working steam engine in the society (as there was when Alexander Hamilton made his remark) or whether there are so many machines in the society that no one, not even the well-placed, can figure out how to find the fuel to run them (as was the case shortly after Richard Nixon made his remark). It is a proposition that is almost true and never works in the long run because it assumes that with knowledge, power, and responsibility a few can determine the best interests of the many. The counter-assumption is that the only way those best interests can be determined, even in a world where knowledge doubles every ten years and $e = mc^2$, is by the many themselves. Which is certainly not to say that a little—or even an average—child shall lead them. Leadership and who can lead within the context of the general welfare as defined by the generality of men is something quite else again. So the third assumption is that men—all the people—given the opportunity for choice will make the best approximation of what is good for them.

Given these three assumptions, how does one get on with the vision-making business? First as to method, I would suggest that there is a useful analogy in the way the common law was created. That law grew out of a series of decisions or choices in particular cases. It rested, in other words, on the assumption that the search for order in the affairs of all men must start from the concern for the plight or condition of a single man. The importance of this point was well stated by Theodore Roosevelt. "While sometimes it is necessary," he wrote in 1900, "from both a legislative and social standpoint, to consider men as a class, yet in the long run our safety lies in recognizing the individuals' worth or lack of worth as the chief basis for action and in shaping our whole conduct, and especially our political conduct, accordingly."

It is in the careful examination of the particular case that one comes closest to an understanding of the blood, sweat, tears, laughter, lupine urges, and natural affections that set the terms for human experience. It is also the place to discover the nature of the actual conflict between the insistent feelings and the unflinchingly rational in man's affairs and to seek accommodation for it.

The concern for the particular case in the creation of the common law was equaled by the interest to proceed through a series of cases toward generality. Accumulating decisions, given increasing shape by the force of precedent, became a sort of controlling synthesis, an accepted regulation for recurring human actions that were similar, if not in detail, in kind. One of the objects of the law was to give continuity and consistency to human affairs, a continuity taken, as Oliver Wendell Holmes said, from experience rather than imposed by the rules of logic. As Lord Wensleydale said, it was "a system which consisted in applying to new combinations of circumstances those rules which we derive from legal principles and judicial precedents."

But as time went on, the new combinations of circumstances, produced by such things as steam power and Maxwell's equations, multiplied in number and intensity. It was then recognized that rules for change were at least as important as rules for stabilizing consistency. Accordingly, the courts were encouraged to invoke not only legal principles and judicial precedents, but the new principle of "public policy." That meant "the prevailing opinion of wise men as to what is for the public good." By this means the courts, still dealing with particular cases, still working within a context supplied by principle and precedent, were given the freedom to search for those changes in decision that would most nearly "suit the changing conditions of society."

Out of this process the common law grew into an organizing context. Sensitive to the claims of every man to appropriate spheres for independent expression and individual action, it yet established norms for the way men must act toward one another and together. The restraining sanctions bore equally upon him whose castle was his home and him whose home was his castle. In its definitions of satisfying human conduct, it became a sort of vision.

It appears that some of the procedures used in the construction of that great system could now be used in the effort to build a larger scheme to fit our future into. The fundamental idea is to start from the particular case. It is almost, but not quite, the poetic notion of trying to find out what God and man is by the careful study of a flower in a crannied wall. The principle, at least, is the same: In the beginning,

think small; don't go after the entire scheme of things head-
on. Such a thought, parenthetically, runs somewhat against
the American grain. We tend to look for the big picture, the
city set on a hill, the great society, the whole long line of the
new frontier, a glory that will transfigure you and me—and
if not soonest at least by tomorrow afternoon.

But the essentials of our present situation seem easier to
get at by the careful formulation and analysis of a well-
selected case—let us say the siting of a power plant—rather
than by the elaboration of some grand design or large-scale
program—let us say Project Independence, 1980—which is
set forth to reassure us that those at the helm know how to
deal with the energy crisis. The siting of a power plant contains such dissimilar but interacting elements as the second
law of thermodynamics, money, the nature of cities, transport, aesthetics, the rights of property, the rights of physical
comfort, geography, greed, the private interest, and the general welfare—to name a few. In this matter, a great many
different kinds of people take an interest—those who make
generators and reactors, those who make and distribute
power, those who use the power distributed to make other
things, those who design rate structures, those who wish to
improve the tax returns, those who breathe the surrounding
atmosphere, those who own property, those who make
power by other means, those who cook, heat, light, and toast
with electricity, and, of course, those who wish to be cooler
than the weather outside.

As things stand now, the various interests that cluster
about the siting and construction of power plants are insufficiently identified and unevenly expressed. The points of
common purpose and of conflict among all these interests are
not clearly revealed. The relative weight to assign to each interest in its collision with the others is not thought through.
Under such conditions, what is momentarily expedient, or

who has doubt, or what is conceived in panic, may well exert
an influence superior to that of some ill-defined sense of the
general welfare or insufficiently informed common sense.
And decisions taken under such influences may contain concealed consequences having to do not only with the contamination of the local air or the short supply of power, but with
land use, property rights, and definitions of citizenship that
could profoundly alter the nature of society.

The problem in the first instance is how to get such a matter as the siting of a power plant defined in such a way that it
can be intelligently analyzed and evaluated in all its parts.
The law uses the adversary process and a cloud of witnesses
who saw things from different angles to formulate a case.
Good trial briefs are simply accurate reconstructions of actual situations. Something of the sort may be done here.
This is the place for Whitehead's philosophers, students, and
practical men to begin their work. Engineers, utility execu-
tives, social scientists, government officials, and "wise men
with a concern for the public good"—a small group—can be
set the task of giving adequate definition to the case of a particular power plant. This definition should include things
like an explanation of need, an examination of cost, descriptions of operating characteristics, identification and consideration of all the interests involved, a statement of probable
consequences for each interest, and a set of alternative solutions for the conflicts of interest discovered. The object of
this process would be to make clear the kind of accommodation—trade-offs—that have to be reached among the parties
at interest—those who need power, those who want money,
those who own property, those who wish to protect the atmosphere, and those who prefer to be cooler than the out-
doors—in order to build a power plant of one kind or another
in one place or another.

In the deliberations of such a group, all parties should have an equal claim to be heard, but principal burdens would fall, no doubt, on two of the parties: those from industry and the philosophers or wise men with a concern for the public good. Those from industry have in their keeping the production of goods and services essential for the development of the technological society. They are the prime movers. The philosophers and wise men are charged with the task of representing the claims of a society that is fit for men to live in. They express the concern for the kind of goods and services offered and the way these goods and services are made. It is in the conflict between these two parties that the nature of the adjustments and trade-offs required to settle a particular case will be most clearly revealed. It is also in this effort at resolution that the collision between the mechanical possibilities and the human necessities—that is, the vexing question of values—will be dealt with.

In this confrontation, it will become obvious that there is more to the anatomy of the body politic than just a bleeding heart or a set of pocketbook nerves. Some accommodation of the requirements of the market and the claims of goodness must be reached, not in the abstract, but within the concrete confines of the particular case. Another way of putting it is to say that while it will never be possible to get away from the test of the market, it should be possible to enlarge the definition of the market so it will include tests for social and human as well as financial solvency.

When the group—a sort of committee of public safety fortified by a staff competent in the assemblage of all the varied, requisite information—has made its formulation of the case, complete with a set of proposed alternatives for sites, capacities, and means of production, the formulation, supported by full explanations, should go before the people in the locality at voting time for a determination among the alternatives. Such exercises, repeated in those different places that may be seeking power plants—New Haven, Topeka, Burlington, and so forth—would in time produce a considerable body of informed opinion on power plants. The resulting information, amplified and modified by repeated experience, collected and codified as in the common law, would produce the evidence necessary to construct some general principles governing the siting and building of economically feasible, mechanically efficient, socially acceptable power plants. The principles would be, in the end, the invention of a variety of people who had different stakes in the game and who understood the nature of the stakes. From these recurring exercises, therefore, would emerge a kind of informed common law for the building of power plants. At that time, the individual exercises could be dispensed with, since those concerned with the building of new plants would have a controlling context to work within.

Power plants have been selected as a demonstration simply because they are on everyone's mind these days, because in the present confused situation, many mistakes have been made, and because they contain, obviously, so many of the elements—mechanical, financial, legal, administrative, social, moral—that enter our present technological situations. But the example of this demonstration can be generally applied in many other critical areas. In transport, communications, the use of natural resources, the organization of production, health care and services, land use, the same elements occur. Indeed, impacted in almost any engineering construct today are all those economic, political, social, and human considerations that men live by or wish they could. Thus, families of cases can be developed in these areas to assist in the passage from the examination of the particular to the framing of general propositions that may govern the proper ordering of the diverse elements in any given situation.

A word more about the formulating groups. They should

serve as ad hoc committees, called into existence to study a particular situation. They should have the means to obtain all the appropriate evidence that bears on their special problem so that they may proceed to their conclusions in an "unflinchingly rational" way and not just by the application of understandings produced by past experience, flashes of intuition, or a special bias. They should meet often enough and long enough to recognize and make some adjustment to one another's information and position. The useful unanimity that must emerge will come not from some compromise worked out by a competent staff, but from individual modifications of position in the interests of the whole. What must end as a statement of agreed-upon policy must start as an educational exercise—learning—and that takes time and what Theodore Roosevelt called the intimacy of actual fights. Such intimacy among all the parties has not been introduced into the making of policies affecting our common welfare in a long time. It suggests, among other things, that the place for such groups to convene is in some neutral corner, and this suggests the universities. Moreover, they are the agencies where the goods and services necessary to support the kind of investigation required are most easily available. And for a third thing, the points at issue—the nature of the problems to be investigated—are the results, in the end, as all technological and social problems are, of the main product line of universities—ideas.

All this is provisionally recognized already by universities. At Harvard, Cornell, Columbia, M.I.T., and Stanford, to name only a few, there are now centers to study the impact of machinery on social organization, to examine policy alternatives, and to worry over the interconnection between the findings of science, the applications of engineering, and the claims of human values. Also, there are in these and many other institutions scholars in growing number who are scru-

tinizing technological man or the post-industrial world or
something called technopolis. What is proposed here is only
a way to take the ideas and understandings that are being developed in the safety of untestable situations, past and
present, and to apply them directly, along with the other interests that have the legitimate claims of "real life," to the
resolution of actual, present, particular cases.

So, what might be expected to come of all this? First, a
scaling down of problems to life size. My friend Captain
Challenger used to say that trying to deal with the Navy
Department was like kicking around a forty-foot sponge.
And that's the way attempts to deal with the world around
us have come to seem to most of us—better leave it to someone with more ambition, or more style, or a better TV presence, or who just happens to be there. But the concentration,
in the beginning, on the particular case—the power plant,
the Northeast corridor—puts the thing in a more manageable
form. Second, it provides a way to engage all parties to a situation—now generally separated by the compartments of
special knowledge or concern—in a common action that will
be carried through to a decision. Third, it offers a quite specific way to improve the learning curve of the man in the
traffic jam who has taken the place of the man in the street.
It presents him with the need for choices—trade-offs—which
is the condition of our world—and supplies the evidence necessary to make sensible choices. Fourth, by extending the
power of choice to him—the vote on the power plant—it re-
covers for him the sense that he can do something about his
situation. Fifth, as the accumulating particular decisions
move toward generality, a context is gradually assembled
within which the parts and pieces and forces of the technological world can be fitted together. Thus assembled, that
context is a product of our intelligence, our experience, our
growing knowledge of, at least, the consequences of our ma-

chinery and our growing understanding of ourselves. Sixth, within such a context, responsible leaders can act with authority to fulfill the obligations implied by the context rather than blunder forward, patching the leakage, damping down the explosions, adjusting to short-falls, amid a welter of minor excitements.

And what have all these nuts and bolts—ad hoc committees, power plants, referenda, useful precedents—got to do with the reenactment of a vision? By way of provisional reply, reference may be made to two other questions which have hung in the air around us for a century. The first, "sublime and terrifying in all its implications," he said, was asked by Thomas Huxley in 1879, "What are you going to do with all those things?" At the time, we did not stay for an answer and it probably was not a good moment to put the question. All the things we then had were not nearly enough to fill up the empty spaces in the vast continent or to satisfy the known needs of the average citizen. What seemed to be wanting then was simply more of the same. Now we are surrounded by such a clutter of things that there is a confusion about how to use them. So, recently there has been much talk about the problem of what to do for the men who have everything. And more recently, that problem has been given sharper focus by the sense that we may not really have the means to sustain what we have already got. Pollution, the shortage of zinc, the energy crisis, these, it turns out, are powerful pedagogical aids. The way to get people to think about a question, apparently, is not to say that its implications in the abstract are terrifying and sublime, but to tell them to set their thermostats to 68°.

So now it seems is a good time to come to terms with Huxley's proposition. How do we plan to make and use our goods and services in a sensible way? If the sky is no longer the limit, what is? The task, obviously, is to establish boundaries to work within. The exercises proposed above are at least one way to get started with the task. They are designed to assist in the construction of a reasonable context within which physical, intellectual, and emotional energy can be organized to serve human needs and interests. They seek to set the limits that may give direction and point to men's actions—as does any vision.

One more word about limits. The thought that any restricting context can be reasonable, that any sort of boundaries can be imposed on growth sets a good many teeth on edge. Industrialists, on the whole, don't like it because it suggests an increase in controls. Economists, on the whole, don't like it because they have huge quantities of intellectual capital invested in and around the concept of growth. The rest of us don't like it because we have been raised in the scheme of great societies where there will always be more for everybody. Besides, the thought seems against all the canons of free enterprise and all the assertions in the Declaration of Independence and also contrary to natural history. From limits to growth it seems all downhill—to the steady state, boredom, impoverishment of the wits, a dying out.

Nobody really knows the truth in these matters. We have just begun to think about the situation. But it may be suggested to the thinkers that the problem before us is only partly biological or economic. It is in part artistic. One half of art is the finding of proper structures—whether the sonata form or a frame of government—within which the raw data of existence can be processed—made intelligible. Given such a context—neither so vague as anarchy nor as specific as a Procrustean bed—the imagination, which abhors the steady state, may proceed, perhaps, indefinitely to novel combinations and interpretations of the data. Indeed, given the proper frame for its exercise, it may turn out to be the one inexhaustible resource that we have.

The second question was put by Lord Bryce in 1888. Brooding upon the excitements of American society ("which they feel to be the work of their own hands"), he asked himself, "What might befall this huge yet delicate fabric . . . [if] all these men ceased to believe that there was any power above them, any future before them, anything in heaven or earth but what their senses told them of; suppose that their consciousness of individual force and responsibility . . . were further weakened by the feeling that their swiftly fleeting life was rounded by a perpetual sleep. . . . Would [then] the moral code stand unshaken, and with it the reverence for law, the sense of duty, toward the community, and even toward the generations yet to come?"

The development of the huge but delicate fabric has reached the point where this proposition has come on for trial. It is assumed here that we—"even we here"—the child, the great beast, the *canis lupus*, the being created in His own image, however one thinks of us—now "hold the power and bear the responsibility." The exercises proposed above rest on the assumption that we—even we here—can find the ways to define that responsibility so that we can build, with our own hands, a world out of our machinery that will be so satisfying that men can afford to think as much of others as of themselves, but with still enough to do so that there is room, within the grand design, for some major excitements. This is an assumption that is not proven, that goes well beyond the available data—which is where the attractive power of any vision lies.

Bibliographical Notes

Sources for Descriptions of Cases

Laommi Baldwin and the Middlesex Canal: George L. Vose, *A Sketch of the Life and Works of Laommi Baldwin* (1885); Lewis M. Lawrence, *The Middlesex Canal* (1942); Christopher Roberts, *The Middlesex Canal, 1793–1860* (1938); manuscripts in the Historical Collections of the Harvard Business School.

John B. Jervis and his several works: Neal Fitzsimmons, ed., *The Reminiscences of John B. Jervis* (1791); John B. Jervis, *Description of the Croton Aqueduct* (1842); *The Question of Labor and Capital* (1877); "A Memoir of American Engineering," *Transactions of the ASCE*, 6 (1878); *Railroad Property* (1881); Letter Collection in Jervis Library, Rome, New York.

John Fritz and the three high rail mill: Joseph Masters, "Brief History of the Early Iron and Steel Industry of the Wood, Morrell and Company and Cambria Iron Company at Johnstown, Pa." (1914), typescript in my possession; John Fritz, *Autobiography* (1912).

W. D. Coolidge and Irving Langmuir and the tungsten lamp: W. D. Coolidge, "Ductile Tungsten," *Transactions of the AIEE*, 29 (1910); "The Development of Ductile Tungsten," in *Sorby Centennial Symposium on the History of Metallurgy*, ed. Cyril, Smith (1965); Irving Langmuir, "Tungsten Lamps," *Transactions of the AIEE*, 32 (1913); "Fundamental Research," *Scientific Monthly*, 40 (1938).

Sources of Background Material for the Study of Cases

Canals: Desmond Fitzgerald, "A History of Engineering in this Country," *Transactions of the ASCE*, 41 (1899); A. Barton Hepburn, *Artificial Waterways and Commercial Development* (1909); Henry W. Hill, *Waterways and Canal Construction in New York State* (1908); Archer B. Hulbert, *The Erie Canal*, Historic Highways of America, vol. 14 (1902), reprinted in 1971.

Ironmaking: Victor S. Clark, *History of Manufacturers in the United States*, 3 vols. (1929); James M. Swank, *History of the Manufacture of Iron in All Ages* (1892); Peter Temin, *Iron and Steel in Nineteenth-Century America* (1964).

Railroads: John H. White, *American Locomotives, 1830–1880* (1968).

The Electric Lamp: Arthur A. Bright, Jr., *The Electric-Lamp Industry* (1949); Percy Dunstreath, *A History of Electrical Power Engineering* (1962); John W. Hammond, *Men and Volts* (1941); Harold C. Passer, *The Electrical Manufacturers, 1875–1900* (1953).

General Works

James Kip French, *The Story of Engineering* (1960); R. S. Kirby, S. Withington, A. B. Darling, F. G. Kilgour, *Engineering in History* (1956); Hans Straub, trans., *A History of Civil Engineering* (1964). Daniel J. Boorstin, *The Americans: The Democratic*

Experience (1973), deals primarily with the social implications of the development of modern engineering, but it examines the course of that development and in so doing makes many points about the nature of the process that are similar to those contained in this book.

Biographies

John T. Broderick, *Welles Rodney Whitney: Pioneer of Industrial Research* (1945); C. B. Stuart, *Lives and Works of Civil and Military Engineers* (1871); David U. Woodbury, *Beloved Scientist* (1944), a life of Elihu Thomson.

Periodicals

The journals or transactions of the American Institute of Electrical Engineers, American Philosophical Society, American Society of Civil Engineers, American Society of Mechanical Engineers, and the Franklin Institute are invaluable not only for their lucid descriptions of particular mechanisms and procedures but as sources, through the years, for enlightenment on the changing state of the various arts and the evolution of an engineering culture. The British journal *Engineering*, containing as it does editorials, essays, excellent drawings and notes on engineering projects all over the world, is especially useful in giving a sense of these changing competences and attitudes.

Index